CONTENTS

Acknowledgements		v
Chapter 1.	**Introduction and overview**	1
	Scope of the review	2
	Terminology	2
	The WHO Developmental Difficulties in Early Childhood Survey	3
	Construction of the survey	3
	Identification of respondents	3
	Limitations of the survey	4
	Outline of chapters	4
Chapter 2.	**Early childhood development and health care systems**	6
	Purpose of chapter and additional key references	6
	Conceptualization of child development	7
	The importance of the early years	8
	The role of the health care system	9
	Summary of research	10
	The role of primary health care	11
	Developmental–behavioural paediatrics	12
	Conclusions and implications for action	13
Chapter 3.	**Epidemiology of developmental difficulties in young children**	14
	Purpose of chapter and additional key references	14
	Conceptualization	14
	Summary of research from LAMI countries	14
	Conclusions and implications for action	17
Chapter 4.	**Developmental risks and protective factors in young children**	18
	Purpose and scope of chapter	18
	Conceptualization of risk and protective factors	18
	Resilience and protective factors	18
	Risk factors	19
	The life-cycle approach to developmental risk factors	20
	Summary of research from LAMI countries	21
	Resilience and protective factors in young children	21
	Risk factors in young children	22
	Conclusions and implications for action	31
Chapter 5.	**Prevention of developmental difficulties**	33
	Purpose of chapter and additional key resources	33
	Conceptualization	34
	A model for preventing developmental difficulties in early childhood	34
	Research in LAMI countries	35

	An exemplary model from a developing country: the WHO/UNICEF Care for Child Development Intervention	38
	Conclusions and implications for action	39
Chapter 6.	**Early detection of developmental difficulties**	**41**
	Purpose of chapter	41
	Conceptualization	41
	Research in LAMI countries	42
	An example from a developing country	47
	Conclusions and implications for action	50
Chapter 7.	**Developmental assessment of young children**	**51**
	Purpose of chapter and additional key references	51
	Conceptualization	51
	Research in LAMI countries	53
	Assessment processes	53
	Assessment instruments	54
	Conclusions and implications for action	57
Chapter 8.	**International classification systems for developmental difficulties in young children**	**59**
	Purpose and scope of the chapter and additional key resources	59
	Conceptualization	59
	The Diagnostic Classification of Mental Health and Developmental Disorders of Infancy and Early Childhood	60
	The International Classification of Diseases	61
	International Classification of Functioning, Disability, and Health	61
	Application of classification systems	62
	Strengths of the classification systems and areas that require improvement	63
	Research in LAMI countries	65
	Conclusions and implications	65
Chapter 9.	**Early intervention (EI)**	**67**
	Purpose and scope of the chapter and additional key resources	67
	Conceptualization	68
	What are EI services?	69
	Who are EI services for?	69
	What major improvements are needed in the conceptualization of EI?	70
	Evidence-based best practices in early intervention	71
	Summary of research in LAMI countries	71
	Important questions for future research	74
	An exemplary model from LAMI countries	75
	Conclusions and implications for action	77
Chapter 10.	**From prevention to intervention: consensus of experts**	**78**
	Advancing policy related to developmental difficulties in early childhood at national levels	78
	Bringing down barriers using common international approaches and platforms	79
	Increasing local capacity by training personnel	79
	Increasing capacity in other specialities related to developmental difficulties	80
	Empowering caregivers	80
	Conducting research	80
References		**81**
Annex 1		**101**

Section 4.
Resources for Survey

28. Please describe the 3 priority actions that you believe would improve EI services in your country in the next 5 years?
    a) ....
    b) ....
    c) ....

29. Please list references for **key publications or web sites** that you have consulted to complete this survey:
    a) ....
    b) ....
    c) ....

30. Please list **key people**, **organizations** or **model programmes** that are related to young children with developmental risks or difficulties in your country:

Name	Contact information (e-mail or web site preferred)
a)	....
b)	....
c)	....

Please provide any further information that you have not been able to provide in the survey and that you would like us to know about young children with developmental difficulties in your country:

Would you like your name to be acknowledged in the final report?
☐ a) No
☐ b) Yes and it should be written as: ....

We greatly appreciate your time and efforts.

ANNEX 1

26. In the following case scenarios, what services would children living **in your area of the country** likely receive? *Please check X in all boxes (a–l) that apply for questions 26.1–26.4.*

		Case Scenarios			
		26.1 Six-month old born prematurely, birth weight 1400 gr, poor weight gain, mild spasticity, not vocalizing	26.2 One-year-old with Down syndrome	26.3 Three-year old with cerebral palsy	26.4 Six-month old whose mother is severely depressed
a)	Healthcare				
b)	Healthcare by same medical doctor				
c)	Sufficient nutrition				
d)	Developmental evaluation				
e)	Hearing evaluation				
f)	Evaluation of vision				
g)	Physical therapy				
h)	Early intervention				
i)	Counseling caregivers on how to support child's development				
j)	Treatment of maternal depression				
k)	Home visits by EI/PT providers				
l)	Financial aid				

27. What is the usual range of hours of *early intervention and physical rehabilitation services* that the following children would qualify to receive in your country?

	Minimum hours/month	Maximum hours/month
27.1 A 12 month old young child has severe cerebral palsy, cognitive and speech and language difficulties		
27.2 A 12 month old child has Down syndrome without medical complications		
27.3 A 6 month old child has birth weight 1000 grams but no obvious developmental difficulties so far		
27.4 A 6 month old child has a mother with severe major depression		

ACKNOWLEDGEMENTS

The World Health Organization wishes to express its deep gratitude to the author of this review, Dr Ilgi Ozturk Ertem, Professor of Pediatrics, Director, Developmental-Behavioral Pediatrics Division, Ankara University School of Medicine, Ankara, Turkey, and visiting professor (2006–2007) at Yale University School of Medicine Department of Pediatrics, New Haven, CT, USA.

The project was led and supervised by Dr Meena Cabral de Mello, Senior Scientist, Department of Maternal, Newborn, Child and Adolescent Health, WHO, Geneva.

This document was reviewed internally by members of the WHO Department of Child and Adolescent Health and the Disability and Rehabilitation Team, and externally by international experts in the field including: Dr Vibha Krishnamurty, Director, Ummeed Child Development Centre, Mumbai, India; Professor Nicholas Lennox, Director, Queensland Centre for Intellectual and Developmental Disability, Brisbane, Australia; Dr Shamim Muhammed, Sangath Organization, Goa, India; Dr Olayinka Omigbodun, Department of Psychiatry, University of Ibadan, Ibadan, Nigeria; Professor Trevor R Parmenter, Director, Centre for Developmental Disability Studies, Sydney, Australia; Professor Atif Rahman, Chair, Department of Child Psychiatry, University of Liverpool, Liverpool, England; Dr Chiara Servili, WHO Eritrea Country Office Asmara (2008); Professor Rune Simeonsson, Professor of School Psychology and Early Childhood Education, University of North Carolina, Chapel Hill, USA; Dr Aisha Yousafzai, Child Health and Disability, Aga Khan University Human Development Program and Aga Khan University Medical College, Department of Paediatrics and Child Health, Karachi, Pakistan, and Dr Nurper Ulkuer, Chief, Early Childhood Development Unit/PDO, United Nations Children's Fund, USA.

Federico Montero and Alana Officer, WHO Disability and Rehabilitation Team, Dr Mercedes de Onis, WHO Department of Nutrition and Dr Tarun Dua, WHO Department of Mental Health provided invaluable comments and suggestions.

Thanks are due to Professor Michael Guralnick (President of the International Society of Early Intervention), Professor David J Schonfeld (past President of the Society of Developmental Behavioral Pediatrics and director of the Developmental Behavioral Pediatrics Division, Cinninnati Children's Hospital), Professor Matthew Melmed (Director of Zero to Three), and Drs John M Levental, Brian Forsyth and Carol Weitzman (Yale University School of Medicine) for their review and comments on the survey, Developmental Difficulties in Early Childhood.

Dr Ertem's consultations with Professor Barry Zuckerman (Chairman of Pediatrics, Boston University School of Medicine, Boston, USA), for this review was supported by a Leadership Development, Fellow's Collaboration grant from Zero to Three. We also thank Zero to Three for providing the gift of an issue of Zero to Three Journal for the respondents of the survey.

Most importantly, we are grateful to the numerous experts around the world for their invaluable contributions to the Developmental Difficulties in Early Childhood Survey. These include:

Argentina: Horacio Lejerraga, MD, Head of Department of Growth and Development. Hospital de Pediatría Garrahan. Buenos Aires, Argentina. hlejarraga@garrahan.gov.ar

Australia: Frank Oberklaid, MD, Professor, Centre for Community Child Health, Royal Children's Hospital, Melbourne, Victoria, Australia. frank.oberklaid@rch.org.au

Bangladesh: Naila Khan PhD, Professor, Child Development and Neurology Unit, Dhaka Shishu (Children's) Hospital, Sher-e-Bangla Nagar, Dhaka, Bangladesh. naila.z.khan@gmail.com

Brazil: Jose Salomao Schwartzman, MD, Professor, Developmental Disorders Postgraduation Program, Mackenzie Presbyterian University. São Paulo, Brazil josess@terra.com.br

Bulgaria: Aneta Popivanova, MD, Assistant Professor of Neonatology, University Clinic of Neonatology, University Hospital of Obstretics and Gynaecology, Sophia, apopivanova@abv.bg

Canada: Emmett Francoeur, MD, Director, Child Development Program and Developmental Behavioral Pediatric Services, Montreal Children's Hospital, McGill University Health Center, Montreal Children's Hospital, Montreal, Quebec, Canada. emmett.francoeur@mcgill.ca

Chile: Paula Bedregal, MD, MPH, PhD, Professor of Public Health, School of Medicine, Pontificia Universidad Católica de Chile, Santiago, Chile, pbedrega@med.puc.cl

China: Jin Xing Ming, MD, Department of Development and Behavioral Pediatrics, Shanghai Children's Medical Center, School of Medicine, Shanghai Jiaotong University, Shanghai 200127, China, zhujing7@public7.sta.net.cn

Egypt : Ala'a Ibrahim Shukrallah MD, Head of Training and Research Unit, Development Support Centre, 30 Haroun St, Geiza, Egypt, alaashuk@yahoo.com

France: Phillipe Compagnon, MD, Hôpital Sainte Thérèse, Bastogne, Belgium philippe.compagnon@wanadoo.fr

Gaza Strip and West Bank: Alam Jarrar, MD, Director, Rehabilitation Program, West Bank and Gaza, Ramallah, Palestine, allam@pmrs.ps

Georgia: Nana Tatishvili, MD, Medical director and head of neurology service, M.Iashvili Central Childrens Hospital, Tbilisi, Georgia. n_tatishvili@mail.ru

India: MKC Nair, MD, Professor of Pediatrics & Clinical Epidemiology Director, Child Development Centre Medical College, Thiruvananthapuram Kerala, India. nairmkc@rediffmail.com

Vibha Krishnamurthy, MD, Director, Ummeed Child Development Center, Mumbai, India. vibha.krish@gmail.com

Indonesia: Anna Alisjahbana, MD, PhD, Professor Emeritus, Founder and Chairperson Surya Kanti Foundation (YSK), "Center for the Development of Child Potentials" Consultant & Advisor, Bandung, Indonesia. alisja_a@melsa.net.id

Israel: Gary Diamond, MD, Director, Child Development Services, Clalit Health Maintenance Organization, Dan Region, Israel, and Vice Director Child Development Institute Schneider Childrens Medical Center of Israel, Petah Tikva, Israel. diamondg@zahav.net.il

Jordan: Saleh Al-Oraibi, PhD, MCSP, Assistant Professor, AL- Hashmite University , Faculty of Allied Health Sciences, Physical Therapy and Rehabilitation Department, Zarka, Jordan, so55@hu.edu.jo

Kyrgyzstan: Nurmuhamed Babadjan, Chief of pediatric rehabilitation department, National Center of Pediatrics. nurmuhamed-babad@mail.ru

Gulmira Nagimidinova, Director of IMCI Center of National Center of Pediatrics and Child Surgery, assistent of department of family medicine of Kyrgyz State Medical Academy, Bishkek, Krygyzstan. nt_gulmira@yahoo.com

Lebanon: Moussa Charafeddine, Vice President Inclusion International, Secretary General Lebanese Parents & Institutional Associations for Intellectually Disabled, President Of MENA Region Inclusion International, President, Friends of Disabled Association-Lebanon, Beirut, Lebonon. moussa@friends-fordisabled.org.lb

Malaysia: Amar Singh HSS, MD, Senior Consultant Paediatrician, Consultant Community Paediatrician Head of Paediatric Department, Ipoh Hospital, Perak, Malaysia. amimar@pc.jaring.my

Pakistan: Zeba A. Rasmussen, Vice Chairman, Chief Executive Officer, Mehnaz Fatima Educational and Welfare Organization, Shahrah-e-Quaid-e-Azam Near Family Health Hospital, Jutial , Gilgit, Pakistan. zebarasmussen@yahoo.com, zeba@comsats.net.pk

Phillipines: Alexis Reyes, MD, Professor, Institute of Child Health and Human Development, University of the Philippines, National Institutes of Health, Manila, Philippines. alexis7591@gmail.com

Romania: Adrian Toma, MD, Chief of the Neonatology Unit, "Panait Sarbu" Obstetrics and Gynecology Hospital, Bucharest, Romania. tomaotiadi@yahoo.com

ACKNOWLEDGEMENTS

Russian Federation: Akaterina Klochkova, PhD, Head of physiotherapy department, St. Petersburg Pavlov Medical University, St Peterburg Early Intervention Institute, St Petersburg, Russian Federation. katya@klo.ioffe.ru

Saudi Arabia: Saleh M. Al Salehi Al Harbi, MD, Medical Director, Children's Hospital, Consultant developmental behavioral pediatrics, King Fahad Medical City, Riyadh, Saudi Arabia, sssnm3@hotmail.com, salsalhi@kfmc.med.sa

Singapore: Rosebeth Marcou, MD, Developmental and Behavioural Paediatrician, Raffles Hospital, Singapore. drmarcou@gmail.com

South Africa: Colleen Adnams, MD, Senior Specialist and Lecturer Head, Developmental (Clinical) Service and Division of Paediatric Neurosciences, Red Cross War Memorial Children's Hospital and School of Child and Adolescent Health, University of Cape Town, South Africa. Colleen.Adnams@uct.ac.za

Turkey: Drs Ilgi Ertem, Derya Gumus Dogan, Bahar Bingoler Pekcici, Ozlem Unal. Developmental-Behavioral Pediatrics Division, Department of Pediatrics, Ankara University School of Medicine, Ankara, Turkey. ertemilgi@yahoo.com

United Kingdom: Val Harpin, MD, Consultant Paediatrician (neurodisability), Ryegate Children's Centre, Sheffield, United Kingdom, val.harpin@sch.nhs.uk

United Republic of Tanzania: Augustine Massawe, MD, Senior Lecturer, Consultant Paediatrician and neonatologist, Muhimbili National Hospital, Muhimbili University College of Health Sciences, Dar es Salaam,Tanzania. draugustine.massawe@gmail.com

United States of America: David J. Schonfeld, MD, Director, Division of Developmental and Behavioral Pediatrics Cincinnati Children's Hospital Medical Center, Cincinnati, Ohio, United States. david.schonfeld@cchmc.org

Viet Nam: Tran Thi Thu Ha, MD, Vice Director of the Rehabilitation Department, National Hospital of Pediatrics, Rehabilitation Director, Hope Center, Hanoi, Vietnam. mdthuha@yahoo.com

For further information about this document please contact Meena Cabral de Mello, Senior Scientist and WHO Focal Person for Early Childhood Development in the Department of Child and Adolescent Health, WHO/HQ, who led and managed this project.

This document is a part of a series of evidence based reviews intended to guide interventions to improve the health, growth and development of children, particularly those living in resource-poor settings. The other reviews of relevance are:

- *A critical link: Interventions for physical growth and psychological development.* WHO/CHS/CAH/99.3 (1999).

- *Family and community practices that promote child survival, growth and development: A review of the evidence.* WHO. ISBN 92 4 159150 1 (2004).

- *The importance of caregiver–child interactions for the survival and healthy development of young children.* WHO. ISBN 924159134X (2004).

- *Mental health and psychosocial well-being among children in severe food shortage situations.* WHO/MSD/MER/06.1 (2006).

- Responsive parenting: interventions and outcomes (2006). *Bulletin of the World Health Organization*, 84:992–999.

- *The role of the health sector in strengthening systems to support children's healthy development in communities affected by HIV/AIDS: A review.* WHO. ISBN 9241594624. (2006).

- *Early child development: A powerful equalizer* (2007). Final Report for the World Health Organization's Commission on Social Determinants of Health. http://www.who.int/child_adolescent_health/documents/ecd_final_m30/en/

- The Lancet: Child development in developing countries series. *The Lancet*, Vol 369 January 6, 2007. http://www.who.int/child_adolescent_health/documents/lancet_child_development/en/index.html

- The Lancet: Child Development 1. Inequality in early childhood: risk and protective factors for early child development. *Lancet* 2011; 378: 1325–38 http://www.thelancet.com/journals/lancet/article/PIIS0140-6736%2811%2960555-2/fulltext.

- The Lancet: Child Development 2: Strategies for reducing inequalities and improving developmental outcomes for young children in low-income and middle-income countries. *Lancet* 2011; 378: 1325–38. http://www.thelancet.com/journals/lancet/article/PIIS0140-6736%2811%2960889-1/fulltext

- *Facts for life*. UNICEF. Fourth edition (2010). ISBN: 9789280644661.

To obtain copies of the above documents and for further information, please contact:

Department of Maternal, Newborn, Child and Adolescent Health
World Health Organization
20 Avenue Appia
1211 Geneva 27
Switzerland

Tel: +41 22 791 3281
Fax: +41 22 791 4853
Email: cah@who.int
Web site: http://www.who.int/child-adolescent-health

Chapter 1

Introduction and overview

The majority of the world's children live in low- and middle-income (LAMI) countries. Often, in these countries, the health care system is the only system that has the potential to reach most young children and their families. For centuries, clinicians, researchers and advocates around the world have been working to prevent, diagnose and treat childhood illness, so that children can enjoy good health and reach adulthood. This task continues to be a challenge. There is still an unacceptable disparity between high-income and LAMI countries with respect to indicators for child survival and health. Equally unacceptable is the disparity between countries in the range of supports available to help children develop optimally, and to prevent, detect and manage developmental difficulties during infancy and early childhood.

Despite long experience in fighting childhood illness and mortality, health care providers in LAMI countries face new challenges in promoting child development. There is, nevertheless, a wealth of information on this topic, generated by researchers and clinicians working in resource-poor conditions. The main premise of the present review lies in the words of the late Professor Mujdat Basaran, a renowned paediatrician in Turkey: "We must generate our own science. We must search and research for information that is pertinent for our own circumstances and we must contribute to the production of the science that will help us move forward." This review therefore compiles the wealth of information that has already accumulated in a systematic framework that can be used by health care providers in LAMI countries.

In this review, the term "developmental difficulties" is used to refer to a range of difficulties experienced by infants and young children, including developmental delay in the areas of cognitive, language, social-emotional, behavioural and neuromotor development. "Early childhood" and "young children" relate to the age range 0 to 3 years. Since economic status is the most important factor determining human

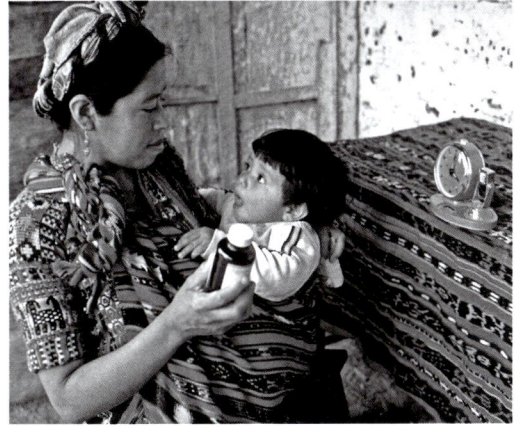

The majority of world's children live in low- and middle-income countries, Nicaragua. © WHO-342031/C.Gaggero

development, countries are categorized as high-income or low- and middle-income according to the World Bank definition (www.siteresources.worldbank.org/DATASTATISTICS/.../CLASS.XLS accessed 21.04.2011).

Developmental difficulties during early childhood are increasingly recognized in LAMI countries as important contributors to morbidity in children and adults. Health care systems in high-income countries provide multiple opportunities for the prevention, early identification and management of developmental difficulties in young children. Interventions to improve the development of young children are becoming increasingly available in LAMI countries, and include low-cost strategies, such as addressing malnutrition and iron deficiency, training caregivers, increasing psychosocial stimulation and providing community-based rehabilitation.

Infancy and early childhood are the best time for the prevention and amelioration of problems that could potentially cause developmental difficulties and affect brain development across the lifespan. A focus on prevention and early intervention for developmental difficulties requires an understanding of the magnitude and nature of the problems, to ensure a match between the interventions delivered and what is needed by the children, their families and their communities.

Many families have contact with the health care system most often – and sometimes only – when their children are young. Health care encounters for young children are, therefore, important opportunities for clinicians in LAMI countries to have a positive influence on development.

In most LAMI countries, the health care system does not have a model for the promotion and monitoring of the development of children, prevention and early identification of risk factors associated with developmental difficulties, and early interventions. Health care providers may not have appropriate knowledge and expertise, and service delivery systems may be inadequate. However, by building local capacity, a systematic approach, specific to the needs of LAMI countries, can be developed. This review seeks to help health care providers and systems in LAMI countries to build such local capacity.

Scope of the review

WHO has previously published three reports related to child development. The first, *A critical link* (WHO, 1999) summarized the importance of addressing both the nutritional and psychosocial aspects of malnutrition and was a seminal report on the need for developmentally based biopsychosocial approaches to child health. The second, *The importance of caregiver–child interactions for the survival and healthy development of young children* (Richter, 2004) contained important information on the most critical component of child development, the relational aspect. The third, *Early childhood development: a powerful equalizer* (Irwin, Siddiqi & Hertzman, 2007), prepared for the WHO Commission on the Social Determinants of Health, provided an in-depth look at the importance of social determinants in shaping child development

This fourth report includes information from low- and middle-income countries on the conceptualization, epidemiology, prevention, detection, assessment and early management of the broad spectrum of developmental risk factors and developmental difficulties in children aged 3 years and under. It does not contain in-depth information on specific developmental risk factors, such as human immunodeficiency virus (HIV) infection and acquired immunodeficiency syndrome (AIDS), low birth weight, malnutrition and chronic illness. This review should not be viewed as a general resource for early childhood disability or for specific developmental disabilities, such as cerebral palsy, genetic or metabolic disorders, autism spectrum disorders, and cognitive or sensory impairments. These topics deserve specific attention beyond the scope of this review. Where relevent and possible, reference is made to other reviews or documents on these topics.

Terminology

During the first three years of life, even children who are showing typical development may be at risk and in need of early intervention services. Children may show differences from the broad range of healthy development without necessarily having a specific disorder or disability. This review includes issues related to a broad spectrum of problems that may affect development. Therefore, the term "developmental difficulty" is used to include conditions that place a child at risk for suboptimal development, or that cause a child to have a developmental deviance, delay, disorder or disability. The term is intended to encompass all children who have limitations in functioning and developing to their full potential, e.g. those living in hunger and social deprivation or born with low birth weight, as well as those with cerebral palsy, autism, cognitive imparments such as Down syndrome, sensory problems, or other physical disabilities, such as spina bifida.

There is no universally accepted definition of developmental pathology during infancy and early childhood (Msall, 2006). "Developmental delay" is often defined as a deviation of development from the normative milestones in the areas of cognitive, language, social, emotional and motor functioning. Neurodevelopmental disorders have been categorized as cerebral palsy, autism, genetic syndromes and metabolic diseases affecting the central nervous system (Batshaw, 2002). Often infants and young children with any kind of difficulty require a broad range of services, referred to as early intervention. While some disabilities merit specified services, there are widely relevant common approaches that can be delivered through health systems for the prevention, early detection and management of developmental difficulties. An in-depth knowledge of the functioning and needs of the child, family and community

> During the first three years of life, even children who are showing typical development may be at risk and in need of early intervention services.

is often more important than the category of the pathology. For this reason, this review adopts a non-categorical approach, as recommended by pioneers in the fields of early intervention and children with special needs (Msall et al., 1994; Msall, 2006; Stein & Silver, 1999; Stein, 2004). This non-categorical approach parallels that of the WHO International Classification of Functioning, Disability and Health for Children and Youth (ICF-CY) framework (WHO, 2007), which is explained in detail in Chapter 8 (Lollar & Simeonsson, 2005; Simeonsson, 2007).

The WHO Developmental Difficulties in Early Childhood Survey

There is little information available about how health care systems are functioning with regard to the prevention, early detection and early management of developmental difficulties. The Developmental Difficulties in Early Childhood (DDEC) Survey was therefore developed to identify the structures and practices in different countries. Sample results from this survey are provided in summary form at the beginning of the relevant chapters in this review. The detailed results will be presented elsewhere.

Construction of the survey

A number of key questions were identified and discussed with a group of experts within the WHO Departments of Child and Adolescent Health and Development, Mental Health, and Nutrition, and the Disability and Rehabilitation Team. In addition, a number of internationally renowned experts in the fields of early childhood development, developmental difficulties and early intervention provided input to and comments on the content and structure of the survey (see Acknowledgements).

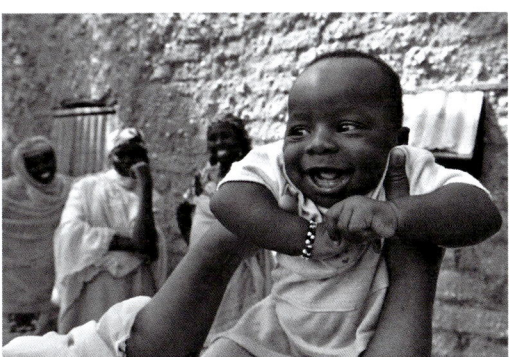

Social interactions begin early in life: 3-month old, Niger.
© UNICEF/NYHQ2009-2569/Holtz

The following WHO projects also informed the construction of the DDEC Survey:

- Atlas: Country Resources for Neurological Disorders (WHO 2004b)
- Mental Health Atlas, (WHO 2005a)
- WHO AIMS: Mental Health Systems in low- and middle-income countries: a WHO-AIMS cross-national analysis (WHO 2005b)
- Atlas: Child and adolescent mental health resources: Global concerns, implications for the future (WHO 2005c)
- Atlas: Epilepsy care in the world (WHO 2005d)
- Atlas: Global resources for persons with intellectual disabilities (WHO 2007b).

A broad literature search was conducted to identify key publications that examined similar constructs. A study conducted by the International Society of Prevention of Child Abuse and Neglect (ISPCAN, 2008) and another of structures and practices of well-child care in ten high-income countries (Kuo et al., 2006) provided useful input to the DDEC.

The reliability of the questions was checked by giving the survey to two expert respondents in each of four countries. When major disagreements were found, questions were removed; for minor disagreements, questions were reworded.

Identification of respondents

The networks of WHO, UNICEF, the Society for Developmental Behavioral Pediatrics, the International Society for Early Intervention and Zero to Three were contacted to identify key experts around the world who met all of the following three criteria.

1. The person was the key expert (or one of the key experts) in the country on early identification, early intervention and rehabilitation of young children aged 0–3 with developmental risks (such as low birth weight or malnutrition) and difficulties (such as developmental delay, cerebral palsy, Down syndrome).

2. The person had in-depth knowledge about the health care system and the training of primary child health care providers in the country. Preference was given to academic paediatricians responsible for training health care providers.

3. The person had good command of English.

A literature search was also conducted to identify professionals who had published on the concepts in the DDEC Survey. When an expert was identi-

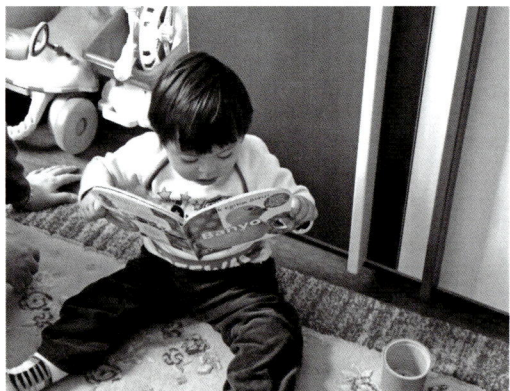

Early stimulation is crucial to optimal development: one-year old with Down syndrome, Turkey. Photo: Canan Gul Gok

fied, at least one of the networks was contacted to confirm that he or she was suitable to be the respondent for the country. In total, experts from 35 countries were identified and invited to participate in the Web-based survey.

Respondents from 31 countries completed the survey, comprising 94% of those identified and eligible. Of these, 6 were from low-income countries, 17 from middle-income countries and 8 from high-income countries. Despite the small number of countries included, the total population of the countries in the survey is approximately 70% of the world population.

Limitations of the survey

There are two main limitations of the DDEC survey – generalizability and reliability. Its generalizability is limited by the fact that countries that were included comprise a portion of the world population. Countries particularly in Africa may not be well represented in this survey. Furthermore, since this survey represents information provided by one expert opinion from each country, the question of reliability and generalizability of the responses remains a limitation. Respondents were knowledgeable, were asked to report about their country as a whole, and to use data and other expert opinions to respond to the questions when possible. However, their views may not reflect the situation in all parts of the country.

Outline of chapters

The body of this review comprises nine chapters. At the beginning of the first eight chapters, the relevant results from the DDEC Survey are given.

Chapter 2 provides a summary of the conceptualization of child development, the importance of the early years and the role of the health care system in ensuring the optimal development of all children. The term "child development" indicates the advancement of the child to reach his or her optimal potential in all areas of human functioning – social, emotional, cognitive, communication and movement. In the past few decades, new imaging techniques have enabled us to visualize how the human brain develops. This chapter summarizes comtemporary theory on early childhood development and provides a framework for why this concept deserves to be addressed in detail within health systems around the world.

Chapter 3 provides a framework for understanding the epidemiology of developmental difficulties in young children by reviewing the existing evidence.

Chapter 4 introduces a conceptual framework, the "Life cycle approach to developmental risk factors", which organizes the risk factors and protective factors for child development in a way that helps countries and communities determine what needs to be done. Research in LAMI countries on preconceptional developmental risk factors that have not previously been fully explored, such as adolescent parenting, unintended pregnancy, inadequate birth interval and consanguinity, are also reviewed.

Chapter 5 provides a new conceptual framework of interventions that can be delivered within the health care system for the prevention of developmental difficulties in young children. Examples of research on prevention in LAMI countries are given, and an exemplary programme, the WHO/UNICEF Care for Child Development Intervention, is summarized.

Chapter 6 deals with early recognition of developmental difficulties in young children. Early recognition allows both preventive and therapeutic approaches to be implemented and is a crucial step in addressing the problems. In high-income countries, the integration of developmental monitoring into health care encounters has been recognized as an important strategy for the early detection of developmental difficulties. This chapter promotes developmental monitoring in LAMI countries, summarizing its conceptualization and addressing key questions of importance for LAMI countries. A novel method of developmental monitoring, which is currently being used in Turkey and which has been specifically developed by the author with attention to the needs of health care providers in LAMI countries, is also introduced. This method is fully complementary with the WHO/UNICEF

Care for Child Development Intervention. When used together, these two methods may provide a systematic, family-centred and strengths-based approach to monitoring the development of young children, to prevent the most common cause of developmental delay (understimulation), to detect developmental difficulties and to provide early intervention.

Chapter 7 focuses on the developmental assessment of young children, to establish a diagnosis, ascertain their level of functioning, determine their needs for additional support and services, and enable them to reach such services. In many resource-rich countries, a team of clinicians from multiple disciplines evaluate the child and the family. In countries with fewer resources, the evaluation of the child may be conducted by one or two clinicians with a less broad experience. The basic principles of developmental assessment, however, can be applied by an experienced clinician in any setting, to give a comprehensive assessment leading to appropriate interventions. This chapter, therefore, provides information on the basic principles of developmental evaluation, the types of developmental assessment that are desirable and how to begin building an infrastructure for such assessments.

Chapter 8 summarizes information on classification systems for developmental difficulties in young children that can be used in LAMI countries. Internationally endorsed classifications facilitate the gathering, conceptualization, interpretation and sharing of information between clinicians and researchers around the world. Countries may also use classifications to determine whether children are eligible for certain services. This chapter places specific emphasis on the WHO International Classification of Functioning, Disability and Health for Children and Youth (WHO, 2007), and provides examples of how this system can be applied to capture the functioning and needs of young children. It also provides a summary of the framework developed by Zero to Three (2005).

Chapter 9 provides a summary of early interventions to guide health care providers and health care policy-makers in LAMI countries in their efforts to improve the lives of developmentally vulnerable children and their families.

Chapter 10 presents the key actions suggested by the respondents to the DDEC Survey. These have been compiled under headings that emerged from a qualitative analysis of the open-ended questions in the survey, i.e. (a) advancing policy related to developmental difficulties in early childhood at national level; (b) breaking down barriers using common international approaches and platforms; (c) increasing local capacity by training personnel; (d) increasing capacity in other specialities related to developmental difficulties; (e) empowering caregivers; and (f) conducting research.

> "…in the context of the successes of current primary health care child survival initiatives, it is essential in low-income countries that increased emphasis be placed on prevention and early identification of developmental disabilities within the primary and maternal and child health care systems. Those systems must in turn be linked to and supported by secondary and tertiary medical services."
>
> *Committee on Nervous System Disorders in Developing Countries, 2001*

Chapter

Early childhood development and health care systems

DDEC Survey results

A number of questions in the DDEC Survey requested information on the infrastructure and role of the health services in addressing developmental difficulties in young children. In most countries, access to health care providers was not an issue. Trained health care providers were either within walking distance or accessible by transportation that was affordable to most of the population. Continuity of health care, however, was a problem. Child development can best be addressed if the same health care provider follows the child over time. In most countries, however, children did not receive primary preventive health care, or care for acute or chronic illness, continuously from the same providers. In most low-income countries, but not high- and middle-income countries, home-visiting was available for the majority of children. In all LAMI countries, there was a shortage of primary health care personnel. General paediatricians, paediatric subspecialists, and professionals trained to deal with children with special needs were also few in number. Although some preservice or in-service training programmes existed, primary health care providers did not generally have the expertise to deal with developmental difficulties.

Purpose of chapter and additional key references

The recent *Lancet* series, "Early childhood development in developing countries", estimated that over 200 million children in developing countries are not reaching their full developmental potential (Grantham-McGregor et al., 2007). The Disease Control Priorities project has stated that 10–20% of individuals have learning or developmental difficulties (Durkin et al., 2006). Developmental difficulties are the most common causes of long-term morbidity (Committee on Nervous System Disorders in Developing Countries, 2001). This chapter summarizes the conceptualization of child development, the importance of the early years of life and the role of the health care system in ensuring optimal development of all children.

In-depth information on the theoretical conceptualization of child development is beyond the scope of this review. Readers are referred to other key documents that contain detailed information on contemporary developmental theories and interventions during infancy and early childhood (Shonkoff & Phillips, 2000; Shonkoff & Meisels, 2003; Guralnick, 2005a; Myers, 1995; Zeanah, 2000; National Scientific Council on the Developing Child, 2007).

The Institute of Medicine has published a book specifically intended to guide health care systems, which reviewed in detail the potential response of such systems to developmental disorders (Committee on Nervous System Disorders in Developing Countries, 2001). Durkin et al. (2006) reviewed the disease burden of learning and developmental difficulties and ways to address these problems.

A number of recent Lancet series – on neonatal survival (Darmstadt et al., 2005; Knippenberg et al., 2005; Martines et al., 2005, Lawn, Cousens & Zupan, 2005), child development in developing countries (Engle et al, 2007; Grantham-McGregor et al., 2007; Walker et al., 2007,), maternal and child undernutrition (Black et al., 2008), global mental health (Barret, 2007; Bhugra & Minas, 2007; Chisholm et al., 2007; Dhanda, 2007; Herrman & Swartz, 2007; Horton, 2007; Jacob et al., 2007; Patel et al., 2007; Prince et al., 2007; Saraceno et al., 2007; Sartorius, 2007; Saxena et al., 2007) and disability (Groce & Trani, 2009; Gottlieb et al., 2009; Trani, 2009) – contain information on addressing developmental difficulties in young children within health care systems.

There are many international resources related to children with developmental difficulties. The United Nations (UN) has two conventions related to children with developmental difficulties: the UN Convention on the Rights of the Child (United Nations, 1989), and the UN Convention on the Rights of Persons with Disabilities (United Nations, 2006). Both affirm that children have the right to develop to their full potential and that countries should guarantee that children with special needs receive the services they require. The second convention promotes and protects the full and equal enjoyment of all human rights and fundamental freedoms by people with disabilities, and is legally binding for all Member States. Article 25 of the Convention requires Member States to ensure access for persons with disabilities to health services that are gender-sensitive, including health-related rehabilitation. However, the Convention does not explicitly define disability. The *UN Standard Rules for the Equalization of Opportunities for Persons with Disabilities*, which was recognized by the UN General Assembly in 1993 (United Nations, 1993), is used for monitoring progress in addressing disability in countries. Importantly, this report addresses the basic preconditions that need to be in place to improve the quality of life of children with developmental difficulties.

WHO has previously published three reports related to child development. The first, *A critical link* (WHO, 1999) documented the critical relationship between the nutritional status of a child and his or her psychological development, and demonstrated the effectiveness of combining interventions to promote early childhood development with efforts to improve child health and nutrition, in an integrated care model. The report highlighted the importance of addressing both the nutritional and psychosocial aspects of malnutrition and was a seminal report on the need for developmentally based biopsychosocial approaches to child health. The second publication, *The importance of caregiver–child interactions for the survival and healthy development of young children* (Richter, 2004) contained important information on the most critical component of child development, the relational aspect. The third, *Early childhood development: a powerful equalizer* (Irwin, Siddiqi & Hertzman, 2007), prepared for the WHO Commission on the Social Determinants of Health, provided an in-depth look at the importance of social determinants in shaping child development. This report highlighted the need for sustained research activities to understand the effects of the environment on biological endowment and early childhood development, and for available evidence to inform actions to further child development social investment strategies at all levels

Conceptualization of child development

The term "child development" indicates advancement of the child in all areas of human functioning: social and emotional, cognitive, communication and movement. A long-standing debate in child development theory relates to the relative influence of nature versus nurture. If nature is assumed to be predominant, child development follows a genetically programmed progression, influenced by biomedical risks. On the other hand, if nurture is considered more important, then the child's development is primarily influenced by the caregiving environment – proximally by the primary caregivers and more distally by the larger community.

The contemporary theoretical conceptualization of child development incorporates the importance of both nature and nurture, parallels the biopsychosocial model of health (Engel 1977), and builds on Bronfenbrenner's bioecological model (Bronfenbrenner & Ceci, 1994). This model postulates that human development takes place through progressively more complex interactions

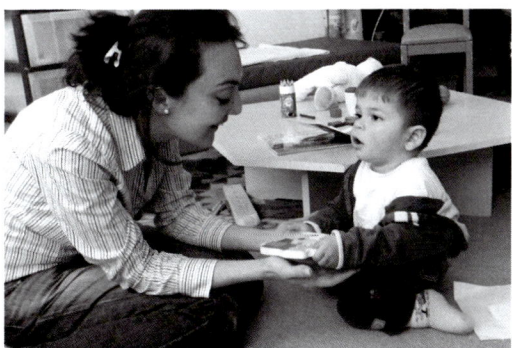

The health system has a key role in monitoring and promoting child development: Developmental Pediatrics Division, Turkey. Photo: Dr. Ilgi Ertem

Figure 1. Conceptualization of child development (reproduced from Ertem, 2011)

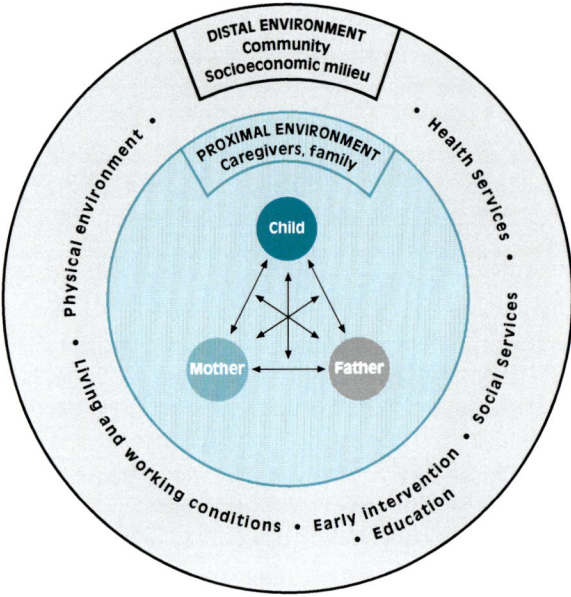

between a "biopsychosocial" human being and the persons, objects, symbols and systems in his or her proximal and distal environment. This interaction is dynamic and the child plays an active role from birth onwards. Figure 1 offers a practical schema for this theory (Ertem, 2011). Here, the biological and genetic endowment of the child is represented by the circle labelled "child". Within this endowment are included concepts such as physical health, temperament, personality, developmental abilities, strengths, coping skills and vulnerabilities. The two other circles, labelled "mother" and "father", represent the equivalent characteristics of each member of the child's proximal caregiving environment – often the parents, but also other key caregivers and siblings. The arrows between the different members signify relationships and interactions between them. The intersecting arrows symbolize how relationships between one pair shape and influence others in the system. The proximal environment includes the child's relationship with the primary caregivers and everyday interactions, such as feeding, comforting, playing and talking. This environment is nested in a community of extended family, neighbours and friends, and a socioeconomic milieu, which includes the workforce, the wealth and well-being of the country, and the health of the population. This distal environment directly or indirectly influences the development of the child, through the living and working conditions of the caregivers, the educational, social and health services, and the physical environment. For example, the child may be affected by the mother or father being stressed because the workplace is not accommodating their needs and desires as new parents. Bioecological theory holds that all components – the biological, psychological, and social functioning of the child and his or her dynamic interactions with the proximal and distal environments – must be addressed when supporting and monitoring child development in primary care. Bronfenbrenner's bioecological perspective offers a useful lens for understanding and supporting young children and their families. This conceptualization can be used in both individual clinical work and in developing model programmes. Bronfenbrenner himself has stressed the importance of recognizing and accepting the uniqueness and strength within each family system and in crafting empowering relations with families (Swick & Williams, 2006).

A more detailed explanation of how distal environments influence child development can be found in the Total Environmental Assessment Model of Early Childhood Development (TEAM-ECD) framework developed for the WHO Commission on Social Determinants of Health (Irwin, Siddiqi & Hertzman, 2007). In the TEAM-ECD framework, there are "spheres of influence" on early childhood development. These spheres are: (1) the individual child, (2) the family and dwelling, (3) residential and relational communities, (4) national, regional and global environments (including global health status, ecological, economic, political and social environments), and (5) early childhood programmes and services. In each sphere of influence, social, economic, cultural and gender factors affect the quality of the proximal caregiving environment, which is instrumental for healthy development in early childhood.

The importance of the early years

The importance of the early years in human development is neither a new nor a Western concept; nor is it, in fact, a concept that is foreign to medical sciences. The works of Avicenna (980–1037), a Persian physician who is considered the father of modern medicine, and Darwin (1809–1882) the founder of the theory of evolution, demonstrate that the concept of early childhood development has occupied the minds of physicians, philosophers, scientists and caregivers for hundreds of years. According to Avicenna, the early years are the most important stage in the life of an individual: "the infant is exposed to problems and difficulties soon after birth and in the early stages of childhood and these influence his psychology and temperament, and hence his moral and ethical development" http://www.ibe.unesco.org/publications/ThinkersPdf/avicenne.pdf accessed 12.07.2007).

Darwin, on the other hand, kept detailed records of the development of his son, providing one of the first systematic studies of child development (Darwin, 1877). A large body of scientific research has been conducted since these early attempts to understand, study and explain child development.

In addition to the bioecological model, two other theoretical concepts – attachment theory and the concept of "the motherhood constellation" – provide guidance on how clinicians can support child development. Attachment theory, developed by Bowlby (1978), suggests that a stable, responsive, nurturing primary relationship enables the child to regulate his or her emotions and develop a secure base from which to explore, learn and form relationships with others. Attachment theory implies that interventions in primary care should address the "caregiver–child" dyad and support parents in helping their infants develop secure attachment. Research in developmental psychology and child psychiatry has shown that a secure attachment to a primary caregiver is associated with healthy emotional and cognitive functioning in later life (Boris et al., 2000). Recent research on children raised in orphanages supports the importance of early relationships and stimulating environments during the early years of life, showing that the cognitive outcome of abandoned children brought up in institutions was markedly below that of abandoned children placed in institutions but then moved to foster care (Nelson et al., 2007).

"The motherhood constellation" is a theoretical construct developed by Stern (1998), a pioneer in infant development and mental health. He refers to the birth of a child and the early years as a specific era of emotional development for the mother. The pregnancy and the birth of the baby change her mental organization, so that her primary preoccupations become keeping the infant alive and protected, caring for the baby so that he or she will become "her" baby and not just any baby (enabling attachment), and creating a supportive, psychologically "holding" environment that supports her mothering. Stern calls this construct "the motherhood constellation".

This construct can help clinicians, who are in fact a component of the holding environment for the mother. Approaches that foster the mother's sense of competence and that empower her will be effective; approaches that criticize her or make her feel inadequate will be counterproductive. A relationship-based, supportive, non-critical, non-didactic approach to parents is the hallmark of many successful interventions.

In the past few decades, new imaging techniques have provided further information on the development of the human brain. Dynamic brain-imaging technology has demonstrated that the full complement of neurons is formed before the third trimester of pregnancy, but that the connections or synapses between these neurons largely develop after birth. This synaptogenesis, and the later "pruning" processes that occur in the developing brain, are constructed to a large degree in the early years within the caregiving environment. The quality of the everyday actions of the parents – smiling, talking, cuddling, singing, and responding to the infant – shapes the circuitry of the developing brain (Shore, 1997; Hannon, 2003).

> Dynamic brain-imaging technology has demonstrated that the full complement of neurons is formed before the third trimester of pregnancy, but that the connections or synapses between these neurons largely develop after birth.

It has also been established that stressors during the early years affect brain architecture. Shonkoff (2006) defines toxic stress as "strong, frequent, and/or prolonged activation of the body's stress-management systems in the absence of the buffering protection of adult support". Precipitants of toxic stress include extreme poverty, recurrent physical or emotional abuse, chronic neglect, severe maternal depression, parental substance abuse and family violence. An important consequence of toxic stress is disruption of the brain architecture, leading to stress-management systems that respond at relatively low thresholds. These low thresholds persist throughout life, increasing the risk of stress-related physical and mental illness throughout childhood and the adult years (Shonkoff, 2006).

The role of the health care system

Many LAMI countries already have the infrastructure needed to support child development within the health care system. For example, India has the world's largest integrated early childhood development services; operational since 1975, functioning in thousands of centres and covering millions of children and mothers, these services aim to improve the health and development of children and families. In 2004, there were 5652 ICDS projects in India, 4533 in rural areas, 759 in tribal areas and 360 in urban areas (Ministry of Women and Child Development, 2009). In Turkey, local health care facilities are located at village level throughout the country, staffed with physicians, nurses and home-visiting midwives. Thus, the health care system in many countries can have a crucial role in promoting child development and in the prevention, early detection and management of developmental difficulties.

The rationale behind this crucial role can be summarized in four key points, as noted below.

1. In any country, the health care system is often the only system that can potentially reach all young children and their families.

2. The biopsychosocial model of child development recognizes that much, if not all, human disease and disability are a function of the interaction between genes and the environment. Physical health and development, though often viewed as separate components of child well-being, are in fact inseparable. The factors that cause poor health, e.g. undernutrition, also affect development. Similarly, factors that cause poor development, e.g. an unresponsive caring environment, also affect health. WHO refers to this as the "critical link" between physical health and psychosocial development (WHO, 1999). Any system intended to address one component, therefore, must be equipped to address both. Often, this system is the health system.

3. Caregivers, families and communities generally have trust in, and contact with, the health care system (Durkin et al, 2006; Committee on Nervous System Disorders in Developing Countries, 2001; Engle et al., 2007). This contact is most frequent when the child is young, for example for immunizations and growth monitoring, as well as for acute and chronic illnesses. Such health care encounters are excellent opportunities to strengthen families' efforts to promote their child's development, and may be the only chance available for professionals in developing countries to positively influence carers of young children and to prevent developmental difficulties.

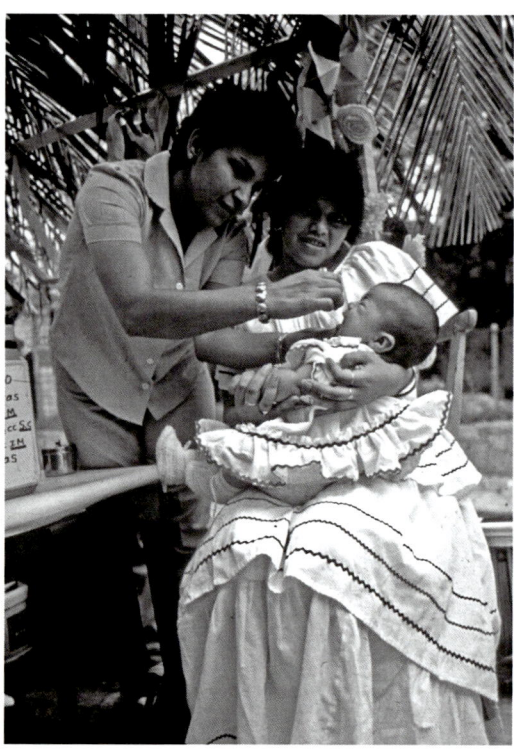

The health system in most countries is the only system that has potential to reach all families. © PAHO/WHO 319032

4. As a result of research showing the positive outcomes of early intervention, there has been particular emphasis in many developed countries on the early identification and management of developmental difficulties within health systems. In most LAMI countries, the personnel and infrastructure for early intervention may not appear to be universally accessible. However, most early intervention programmes for young children with developmental difficulties do not require extensive staffing, and work best when administered through caregivers. The training of caregivers in early intervention is feasible in LAMI countries. As the availability of early intervention and community-based rehabilitation increases, the need for the early detection of problems through the health care system is becoming more evident.

Summary of research

Research in high-income populations has shown that promotion of development in paediatric health care encounters has many potential benefits for children and families. For decades, high-income countries have included within the health care system efforts to promote child development. These countries have also mainstreamed the early detection of developmental difficulties and links to early intervention services. This placing of health care delivery in a developmental context has benefits for both physical health and development. This is especially attractive where developmental approaches are added to existing structures in routine primary care. There are many examples in high-income countries of how a developmental approach has been incorporated into primary care for young children (Regalado & Halfon, 2001). These include Sure Start in England (Roberts & Hall, 2000), the European Early Promotion Project which has taken place in eight countries (Roberts et al, 2002), Help me Grow (Dworkin, 2006), Bright Futures (Green, 1994; Hagan, Shaw & Duncan, 2008; Knight, Frazer & Emans, 2001), Healthy Steps (Niederman et al., 2007; McLearn et al., 2004; Minkovitz et al., 2001; Zuckerman et al., 1997), Reach Out and Read (Needleman et al.,1991), and Touchpoints in the United States (Brazelton, 1999; Hornstein, O'Brien & Stadtler, 1997). In addition, research has focused on the early detection and management of developmental difficulties (Council on Children with Disabilities, 2006).

Child mortality and morbidity patterns in LAMI countries are changing dramtically. In most countries, childhood mortality has declined considerably in the past 20 years. The major causes of death have also changed. For example, in Bangladesh, chronic diseases and injuries have overtaken infectious diseases as the leading causes of child death (Rahman et al., 2004c). Further research is needed in LAMI countries to understand these changes and improve the planning of appropriate policies to address the new challenges.

The role of primary health care

Primary health care providers are in a key position to address child development in developing countries. Often they are the only service providers who reach young children and their families, and they are generally trusted in their communities. In addition, their background enables them to identify and take action against the biological and psychosocial causes of developmental difficulties.

The DDEC Survey found that, in most of the countries, health centres were readily accessible to the majority of the population. Home-visiting by health providers – an important vehicle for integrating child development concepts into health care delivery – was also routinely practised in many of the LAMI countries. Accessibility is one of the features of the health system that make it so important in addressing child development issues in LAMI countries.

There are, however, many potential barriers in the primary health care system that can make this task difficult. Continuity of care – receiving health care from the same provider over a period of time – is one of the most important principles and is crucial to the delivery of developmentally appropriate health care. In the continuity-of-care model, each child (and sometimes family) is followed over time by the same health care provider. Studies in the United States during the 1970s showed the beneficial effects of receiving continuous health care from the same provider (Alpert et al., 1976; Gordis & Markowitz, 1971; Starfield et al., 1976). The benefits of continuous primary care over episodic care included: fewer hospitalizations, operations, visits for illness, and breaking of appointments; more health supervision visits, use of preventive services, and patient satisfaction; and lower costs (Alpert et al., 1976). Since the 1980s, developed countries have tried to ensure that each child has a continuous primary health care provider. More research is needed on the effects of continuity of care in LAMI countries and the changes to the system that would be needed to ensure such continuity.

> Primary health care providers are in a key position to address child development in developing countries. Often they are the only service providers who reach young children and their families, and they are generally trusted in their communities.

The quality of the support given by the health care provider will depend on his or her training and experience in child development concepts. The DDEC Survey indicated that health care providers, particularly in the LAMI countries, generally do not have adequate training and experience in the prevention, early detection and management of developmental difficulties in young children. The limited research from LAMI countries also indicates that primary health care clinicians require training in counselling caregivers on child development and detecting and managing related difficulties (Powell et al., 2004; Rahman et al., 2004a, 2008; Turmusani, Vreede & Wirz, 2002; Walker et al., 2005; WHO, 1999, 2001a, 2006). WHO and UNICEF have developed a number of resources to help train clinicians in LAMI countries to address child development. Community-based rehabilitation (CBR) interventions promoted by WHO for the past 20 years, for example, are becoming available for young children in developing countries (Beard, 2007; Lozoff, Jimenez & Smith, 2006; Richter, 2004). WHO/UNICEF training modules on "Care for child development intervention" (see Chapter 5 for more information) have been available as a component of Integrated Management of Childhood Illness (IMCI) (WHO, 2001a) and currently as an intervention that can be integrated into processes other than IMCI (WHO, 2001c). WHO has also incorporated child development messages in the training materials for the newly launched WHO growth standards (Borghi et al., 2006; de Onis et al., 2007). WHO and UNICEF are continuing to work on incorporating a developmental approach in primary health care.

Because of the small amount of research on feasible models in developing countries, there is limited information on what needs to be done to integrate these actions and interventions into health providers' practices, and whether they are effective. Studies from Brazil (Figueiras et al., 2003), India (Bhatia & Joseph, 2000; Kalra, Seth & Sapra, 2005), Singapore (Lian et al., 2003) and Turkey (Ertem et al., 2009) have highlighted deficits in the knowledge of primary health care providers in this area. Three studies from developing countries have shown promising results in training clinicians to address specific areas including identification of developmental disabilities (Mathur et al., 1995; Wirz et al., 2005), promotion of parenting skills and psychosocial stimulation (Powell et al., 2004), and counselling caregivers on promoting child development during visits for acute minor illness (Ertem et al., 2006). These studies, however, provide limited information, since each focuses on only one aspect of child development training and examines the efficacy of training under controlled research conditions. More research and information are needed from developing countries on the effectiveness and sustainability of comprehensive models for addressing child development within health care systems.

Developmental–behavioural paediatrics

As a guide to progress in the area of developmental disorders, the US Institute of Medicine released a report in 2001 (Committee on Nervous System Disorders in Developing Countries, 2001), which recommended that "in the context of the successes of current primary health care child survival initiatives, it is essential in low-income countries that increased emphasis be placed on prevention and early identification of developmental disabilities within the primary and maternal and child health care systems. Those systems must in turn be linked to and supported by secondary and tertiary medical services." All levels of services should also be linked to disciplines that can create the knowledge base for the incorporation of child development concepts within health systems. Developmental–behavioural paediatrics has for decades pioneered the introduction of concepts of child development within health systems (Friedman, 1970, 1975; Haggerty & Friedman, 2003; Richmond 1967; Shonkoff & Kennell, 1992; Shonkoff, 1993; Venter, 1997b; Shonkoff & Phillips, 2000; Shonkoff & Meisels, 2003; Shonkoff, 2006). This field has been cross-fertilized by paediatrics, child psychology, child development, early intervention and other related disciplines, and thus combines the disciplines of paediatrics, child health and child development. The exact number and distribution of developmental–behavioural paediatricians around the world is unknown. In the DDEC Survey, 55% of respondents identified themselves as developmental–behavioural or developmental paediatricians. In some countries, such as Turkey and India, small-scale training programmes have been started, to establish tertiary centres to train further leaders. There is an urgent need to promote developmental–behavioural paediatrics internationally, to develop training programmes for paediatricians, and to share information between clinicians, academicians, and researchers around the world.

> "...in the context of the successes of current primary health care child survival initiatives, it is essential in low-income countries that increased emphasis be placed on prevention and early identification of developmental disabilities within the primary and maternal and child health care systems. Those systems must in turn be linked to and supported by secondary and tertiary medical services."
>
> *Committee on Nervous System Disorders in Developing Countries, 2001*

Conclusions and implications for action

1. The development of the cognitive, social-emotional, language and movement functions of the young child is influenced by the biological endowment and health of the child, as well as by the relationships with the primary caregivers, family, and support systems in the community. The early years of life are a period of maximal growth and development of the human brain and are therefore extremely important in determining whether the person reaches his or her full potential.

2. In most countries, the health care system is the only system that has the potential to reach all young children and their families. It therefore provides an excellent opportunity to address child development as well as physical health – two inseparable aspects of the well-being and productivity of the child and later adult.

3. There is an unacceptable disparity between high-income and low- and middle-income countries with respect to the range of supports provided to optimize child development and prevent and manage developmental risks and difficulties.

4. A roadmap is needed for health care systems in LAMI countries to guide their efforts to address child development. There is a wealth of information, from high-income countries as well as from the LAMI countries themselves, regarding the development of young children. On this basis, countries should be able to develop and adopt cost-effective, sustainable interventions to address the development of young children through the health care system.

5. The lack of availability of continuous care, inadequate training and experience of health care providers and insufficient secondary- and tertiary-level health centres that can provide support to primary health care workers in dealing with developmental difficulties appear to be major barriers.

6. There is a need for training of subspecialists in LAMI countries in developmental–behavioural paediatrics and allied disciplines, so that they can then train front-line primary health care providers in concepts related to child development and related difficulties.

7. Research and evidence on sustainable models and programmes that address child development and developmental difficulties in LAMI countries are greatly needed.

Chapter 3

Epidemiology of developmental difficulties in young children

DDEC Survey results

The DDEC Survey included one question (see Annex 1, question 13) about the epidemiology of developmental difficulties in young children. In 25 countries (81%), there had been no epidemiological studies in the past ten years that provided specific information on children aged 0–36 months with developmental difficulties. In the six countries (19%) where there had been such surveys, the prevalence of developmental difficulties in young children ranged from 5% to 12%.

Purpose of chapter and additional key references

Epidemiological information about a disease or disorder is crucial to determine the need for services. This chapter provides a framework for understanding the epidemiology of developmental difficulties in young children by reviewing the existing evidence. There has been very little specific research on the epidemiology of developmental difficulties in children aged 3 years and under. Key resources include Durkin et al. (2006), the Committee on Nervous System Disorders in Developing Countries (2001), Maulik & Darmstadt (2007), and the *Lancet* series on disability (Gottlieb et al., 2009).

Conceptualization

Epidemiological studies use two parameters to report on the occurrence of a disorder in a given population: incidence and prevalence. Incidence is the frequency of newly occurring cases each year, while prevalence is the number of cases in a population at a point in time. Because incidence rates are independent of survival rates, they provide more information on etiology. However, determining the incidence of developmental difficulties in children is difficult, because the onset is often insidious and the disorder becomes recognizable only later. Furthermore, true incidence can rarely be determined, as only a minority of the severe forms of developmental difficulty survive long enough to be identified (Hook, 1982).

In high-income countries, epidemiological studies have generally relied on cross-sectional methods and service registries to measure prevalence. In the United States, one study showed that 13% of children aged 3–17 years had a developmental disability (Boulet, Boyle & Schieve, 2009). Previously, a national survey in 1988 found that 17% of children aged 0–17 years had had a developmental disability (Boyle, Decoufle & Yeargin-Allsopp, 1994). In LAMI countries, where registries are often not available, information on the prevalence of developmental difficulties and their impact is insufficient and often unreliable. A recent review by Maulik & Darmstadt (2007) found that most studies of developmental disabilities in children in developing countries that have been published in peer-reviewed journals were concerned with the epidemiology of the disorders. Nevertheless, it remains difficult to ascertain the prevalence of developmental difficulties in young children in LAMI countries for three reasons:

a) the studies conducted did not meet appropriate quality standards;

b) they used different definitions of developmental difficulties;

c) they used different instruments to detect developmental difficulties.

Summary of research from LAMI countries

Survey tools that aim to determine the prevalence of developmental difficulties in resource-poor countries, such as the WHO tool for neurological impairments (Mung'ala-Odera & Newton, 2007) and the "Ten Questions Questionnaire"

(Durkin, Hasan & Hasan, 1995; Gottlieb et al., 2009; Mung'ala-Odera et al., 2004; Thorburn et al., 1992) have been adapted from adult questionnaires and have been shown to identify only children with severe disabilities (Mung'ala-Odera & Newton, 2007). The true prevalence of developmental difficulties in children aged 0–3 years is unknown. In the recent *Lancet* series on disability, Gottlieb et al. (2009) determined the percentage of children screening positive for, or at risk of, disability in Multiple Indicator Cluster Surveys (MICSs) carried out in 18 countries in 2005–2006. The MICS used the "ten questions" screen to identify disability in household surveys. The analysis found that a median 23% (range 3–48%) of children aged 2–9 years screened positive for disability (Gottlieb et al., 2009).

Apart from household surveys, studies in LAMI countries to determine rates of developmental difficulties have used rural participatory appraisal (Gona, Hartley & Newton, 2006; Kuruvilla & Joseph, 1999), key informant method (Muhit et al., 2007) and identification of disability by schoolchildren (Saeed et al., 1999). The "Ten Questions Questionnaire" was not designed to detect children with mild to moderate difficulties, such as social and emotional problems but rather, it focuses on more obvious signs of disability, particularly in older children including hearing and visual impairments. Some authors have speculated that, while the overall prevalence of disability in LAMI countries has remained constant over the past ten years, there has been a shift from more severe disabilities to milder problems related to cognitive impairment, behavioural problems, hearing and communication impairments (Khan et al., 2006). The commonly used screening tools may not adequately detect these difficulties.

Despite the lack of conclusive information on the prevalence of developmental difficulties in LAMI countries, it is known that these disorders constitute a great proportion of childhood morbidity and are a public health problem in all countries (Mung'ala-Odera & Newton, 2007). In the United States, it is estimated that 10–20% of children have developmental difficulties (Benedict & Farel, 2003; Boyle, Decoufle & Yeargin-Allsopp, 1994). Because LAMI countries have higher rates of risk factors that affect young children's development, such as poverty, malnutrition and related deficiencies, intrauterine growth retardation, chronic illness and deficiencies in psychosocial stimulation, the prevalence of developmental difficulties is almost certainly higher than in high-income countries (Committee on Nervous System

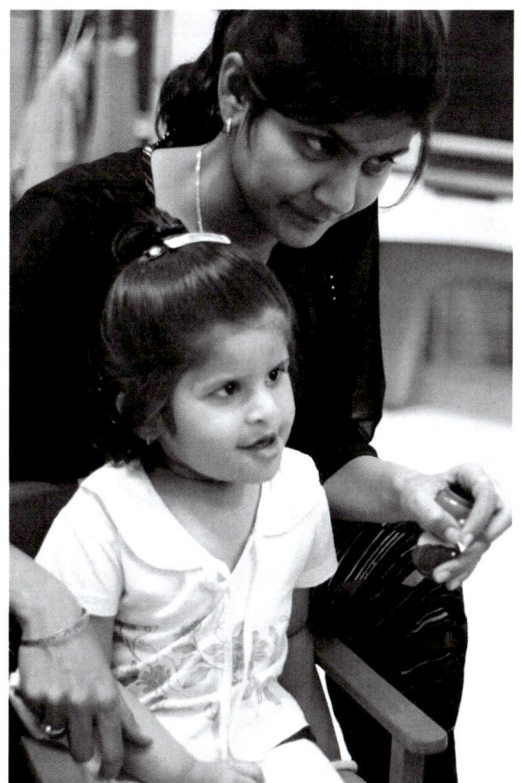

Developmental difficulties are common in early childhood: child and caregiver during early intervention, India. Photo: Dr. Vibha Krishnamurthy

Disorders in Developing Countries, 2001; Durkin et al., 2006; Grantham-McGregor et al., 2007).

Rates of developmental difficulties in young children published in peer-reviewed journals have been inconsistent, ranging from a low of 3.5% in Ethiopia to a high of 24% in Brazil, mainly because of differences in definitions (Abiodun, 1993; Ashenafi et al., 2000; Al-Hazmy, Al Sweilan & Al-Moussa, 2004; Anselmi et al., 2004; Bendel et al., 1989; Diop et al., 1982; Eapen, Zoubeidi & Yunis, 2004; Srinath et al., 2005; Yaqoob et al., 2004) (Table 1). In most of the studies, however, one would expect that the prevalence rates would be higher. One explanation for the low prevalence rates found is that most of the studies relied on caregiver reports of disability and questionnaires such as the "ten question" screen, which were designed to detect severe disability in older children. Fear of stigmatization, lack of trust in treatment or interventions, and uncertainty about what constitutes normal development may have led caregivers to underestimate the developmental difficulties.

The first comprehensive nationwide prevalence study in Israel showed a prevalence of chronic conditions and illnesses causing disability of

Table 1. Epidemiology of developmental difficulties

Country (author, year)	Number	Age (years)	Prevalence (%)	Definition of developmental difficulty used in study
Brazil (Anselmi et al., 2004)	624	2–3	24	Behavioural problem
Senegal (Diop et al., 1982)	545	5–15	17	Emotional/mental health problem
Nigeria (Abiodun, 1993)	500	5–15	15	Psychiatric morbidity
India (Srinath et al., 2005)	2 064	0–16	12.5	ICD-10 diagnosis of mental or psychiatric disorder
United Arab Emirates (Eapen, Zoubeidi & Yunis, 2004)	694	2–3	10	Language delays
Israel (Bendel et al., 1989)	9 854	2–3	8.9	Developmental delay/disability
Saudi Arabia (Al-Hazmy, Al Sweilan & Al-Moussa, 2004)	60 630	0–16	6.3	Disability
Pakistan (Yaqoob et al., 2004)	1 476	12	6.2	Mild mental retardation
China (Sun et al., 2003)	78 000	0–7	5.6	Vision, mental, hearing, language, psychiatric and motor
Saudi Arabia (Milaat et al., 2001)	3 733	0–15	3.7	Wide range of disability
Ethiopia (Ashenafi et al., 2001)	1 477	0–15	3.5	Mental/behavioural problem

8.9% in approximately 10 000 Israeli Jewish children aged 2–3 years (Bendel et al., 1989). A population-based survey of childhood disability in Saudi Arabia, using the "ten questions" tool (Milaat et al., 2001), found a prevalence of 3.7%. In China, approximately 78 000 children aged 0–7 years were tested to determine the prevalence of vision, mental, hearing, language, psychiatric and motor problems. The prevalence of all disabilities was found to be 5.6 per 1000; mental disorders and language problems had the highest prevalence (1.88 per 1000) (Sun et al., 2003). An epidemiological survey covering all regions of Saudi Arabia included 60 630 children under 16 years of age; the prevalence of "handicap" was 6.3% (Al-Hazmy, Al Sweilan & Al-Moussa, 2004). The prevalence of mild intellectual disability in Lahore, Pakistan, was found to be 6.2% (Yaqoob et al., 2004). The prevalence of behavioural problems in 3-year-old children screened with the Child Behavior Checklist (CBCL) for ages 2–3 in the United Arab Emirates was 10% (Eapen, Zoubeidi & Yunis, 2004). In an epidemiological survey in Bangalore, India, the prevalence of mental and psychiatric disorders among 0–16-year-old children was found to be 12.5%. The rate among children aged 3 years and under was 13.8%, with breath-holding spells, pica, behaviour disorders, expressive language disorder and mental retardation the most common diagnoses (Srinath et al., 2005). In a UNICEF-supported study in Pattanakkad rural block, Kerala, India, the prevalence of development delay, deformity, and disability among children aged 5 years and under was reported as 2.5%; the prevalence of developmental disabilities up to 2 years of age was found to be 2.3% (Nair et al., 2009). Interestingly, in the same study, the prevalence of speech and language-related difficulties in children was found to be 29.8%. In rural Nepal, the population prevalence of disability was reported to be 0.95% (Sauvey et al., 2005).

In summary, the prevelance rates of developmental difficulties in young children differ between studies, mainly as a result of differences in research methodology and definitions of disability. Because of the considerably higher rates of risks for child development, the Disease Control Priorities in Developing Countries Project concluded that significantly more children in

> Because of the considerably higher rates of risks for child development, the Disease Control Priorities in Developing Countries Project concluded that significantly more children in LAMI countries will experience developmental difficulties than in high-income countries.

LAMI countries will experience developmental difficulties than in high-income countries (Durkin et al., 2006). Given that 10–20% of children in high-income countries experience developmental difficulties, the burden for children and families in developing countries can be appreciated. For this reason developmental difficulties deserve serious attention as one of the disease control priorities for developing countries.

Conclusions and implications for action

1. The prevalence of developmental difficulties during early childhood is high in all countries. Around the world, these conditions are more common than any other chronic condition that results in major morbidity across the lifespan. In countries with a high prevalence of risk factors that adversely affect early childhood development (such as malnutrition, infectious disease epidemics, iron deficiency and low birth weight), the rates of developmental difficulties can be expected to be high. Developmental difficulties should thus be a priority in LAMI countries.

2. Research on the epidemiology of developmental difficulties in LAMI countries over the past 30 years has not provided conclusive evidence on the prevalence of developmental difficulties. The research has been subject to methodological flaws, including reporting bias and inconsistencies in the definition and detection of developmental difficulties.

3. It is recommended that international standards and common approaches be formulated for definitions, population-based methods of detection of developmental difficulties, and the key research constituents to ensure the production of scientifically valid evidence.

4. Studies on prevalence are difficult to conduct in LAMI countries. There is already sufficient evidence that the prevalence of developmental difficulties in young children is high enough to warrant widespread prevention and intervention efforts in all countries. Provision of services to prevent and manage such difficulties should not be constrained by lack of data on epidemiology.

Chapter 4

Developmental risks and protective factors in young children

DDEC Survey results

Questions in the DDEC Survey that pertained to risk factors requested information on the proportion of health care providers likely to have experience and training in identifying developmental risk factors in young children (see Annex 1, questions 4.1 and 4.2). In less than half of the countries (45%), most health care providers had some training and experience in using interview and observational skills to identify biological risk factors, such as low birth weight. More strikingly, in only 12% of the countries had most health care providers had training and experience in using interview and observational skills to identify social and emotional risk factors, such as maternal depression.

Purpose and scope of chapter

This chapter introduces a conceptual framework for viewing the factors that impede or facilitate child development. A comprehensive consideration of each risk and protective factor is beyond the scope of this review. Emphasis is therefore given to risk factors that have not been reviewed in other documents, and readers are referred to other key publications for further information.

Conceptualization of risk and protective factors

Until recently, in LAMI countries, interventions to improve child survival took precedence over those to address child development. Child survival, physical health and development, however, are inseparable components of well-being. Every condition that poses a risk for child survival may also be a risk factor for child development. Conversely, factors that threaten child development may also be risks to survival.

A conceptual framework of risk and protective factors is important for addressing child development and developmental difficulties in health systems in LAMI countries. Without such a framework, risk factors that affect child development may be overlooked, together with the interventions to address them. This chapter summarizes concepts such as resilience, protective factors and risk factors, and introduces a new conceptualization related to developmental risks, the "life cycle approach".

Resilience and protective factors

Many children who experience adverse conditions during their early years grow up to become healthy and functioning adults. Rutter defines resilience as "an interactive concept that refers to a relative resistance to environmental risk experiences or the overcoming of stress or adversity" (Rutter, 2006). Resilience differs from general concepts of risk and protective factors, in that it incorporates factors specific to each individual that enable him or her to overcome adversity. Studies on resilience date back to the 1960s, when Werner and colleagues started to follow the entire birth cohort of 698 infants on the Hawaiian island of Kauai (Werner, 1992). This study, which lasted 30 years, demonstrated that children exposed to risk factors (for example, premature birth coupled with an unstable household and a mentally ill mother) experienced more problems with delinquency, mental and physical health, and family stability than children exposed to fewer risk factors. However, many high-risk children displayed resilience and developed into healthy, happy adults despite their problematic histories. Werner and colleagues identified protective factors that may have counterbalanced the risk factors. Important protective factors were a strong bond with a caregiver other than the parents (such as an aunt, babysitter, or teacher) and involvement in a community group.

Since the Kauai study, research on resilience

has grown, providing an increased understanding of child development that can directly influence interventions. Research on child-related resilience factors has long included psychological, behavioural and social aspects; more recently, with advances in neuroscience, neurobiological mechanisms of resilience, including neural plasticity, neuroendocrinological pathways and gene–environment interplay, are also being studied. New concepts, such as "maternal optimism" (Jones et al., 2002), are being added to more traditional caregiver-related concepts, such as maternal sensitivity and responsiveness (Conway & McDonough, 2006). Environmental factors, such as poverty, are still key components of research on resilience.

Early experiences of stress and adversity may affect neural structures, resulting in constrained resilience (Rutter, 2006). Resilience is often regarded as relating to innate qualities residing in individuals. Examples of these qualities are behavioural and emotional self-regulation, characteristic of optimal mental health, and cognitive self-regulation, characteristic of high intelligence. Such qualities have been shown to contribute to the mental health and academic achievement of children. Nevertheless, research has also shown that these individual qualities may not suffice to overcome the effects of environmental challenges, such as poor parenting, antisocial peers, low-resource communities, and economic hardship. For example, research on children who were adopted after living in orphanages has shown that, although there is "catch up" in their cognitive and social emotional development, those adopted later had lower "catch up" (O'Connor et al., 2000). Sameroff & Rosenblum (2006) state that "the effects of single environmental challenges become very large when accumulated into multiple risk scores, even affecting the development of offspring in the next generation". Research also indicates that child and family protective factors in early childhood are significantly associated with positive adjustment in later years (Vanderbilt-Adriance & Shaw, 2006). The characteristics of a child's caregiving system, emotionally responsive, competent parenting, and caregiver resources, such as education, mental health, and relational history, are direct proximal predictors of resilience in children (Wyman et al., 1999).

Resilience and protective factors are discussed at more length in a special volume of the *Annals of the New York Academy of Sciences* (Lester, Masten & McEwen, 2006).

> **Early experiences of stress and adversity may affect neural structures, resulting in constrained resilience. Resilience is often regarded as relating to innate qualities residing in individuals.**

Risk factors

Four different approaches have been used to conceptualize risk factors for development of young children.

1. A common approach has been to divide risk factors into biological and psychosocial risks, as was done in the *Lancet* series, "Child development in developing countries" (Walker et al., 2007). While this approach is a major advance on considering only biomedical risks, it is important to remember that risks often: (a) have both biomedical and psychosocial pathways; (b) occur together; and (c) must be managed using interventions that include both biological and psychosocial components. For example, iron deficiency has an adverse impact on child development through a biological pathway (Lozoff & Georgieff, 2006; Lozoff, Jimenez & Smith, 2006) and may be described as a biological risk. The causes of iron deficiency, however, are embedded in psychosocial risks, such as poverty, maternal iron deficiency and low maternal intelligence and education level (Wachs et al., 2005). Furthermore, iron deficiency negatively affects mother–child interactions through a psychosocial pathway (Corapci, Radan & Lozoff, 2006). Another example is maternal depression, which has been considered a psychosocial risk because of its effects on mother–child interactions and child attachment patterns (Campbell et al., 2004; Cicchetti, Rogosch & Toth, 1998; Currie & Rademacher, 2004). Research has also shown that children of mothers who are depressed experience illness more frequently than other children (Patel, DeSouza & Rodrigues, 2003; Rahman et al., 2004a). Thus, a psychosocial risk factor may have a biomedical pathway as well as a psychosocial one. Biological and psychosocial risks often occur together. For example, children born prematurely (biological risk) are often born to mothers with low education levels, living in poverty (psychosocial risks). This phenomenon has been referred to as the "double jeopardy" (Parker, Greer & Zuckerman, 1988). An individual child may

have a number of risk factors at a given point in time or may encounter multiple risk factors over the course of his or her development. In both situations, the effects are cumulative and detrimental to the development of the child.

2. A second approach to risk factors is categorical; this is exemplified in the Disease Control Priorities Project (DCPP) in Developing Countries (Jamison et al., 2006), in which risks for learning and developmental disabilities were categorized as: genetic; multifactorial (e.g. genetic and nutritional, such as neural tube defects); nutritional; infections; toxic exposures; maternal disorders; perinatal complications (such as brain injuries associated with premature birth or birth asphyxia); injuries; economic disadvantage; social and cognitive deprivation; and unknown causes. This categorization is useful as a way of viewing potential causes of developmental difficulties, but does not provide a framework for recognizing when risk factors co-occur and when to intervene. Also, risk factors that fall outside of the specified categories, such as unintended pregnancy and adolescent parenting, may be overlooked.

3. The *Diagnostic Classification of Mental Health and Developmental Disorders of Infancy and Early Childhood Revised Edition* (DC 0-3R) (Zero to Three, 2005) provides yet another conceptualization of developmental risks. In the DC 0-3 R, which is described in detail in Chapter 8, risk factors are referred to as "psychosocial and environmental stressors". It is emphasized that four components determine the impact of any risk: (a) the severity; (b) the duration; (c) the developmental level of the child when he or she is exposed to the risk; and (d) the coping ability and capacity of the caregivers. While the list of stressors (risk factors) is exhaustive, it is designed for clinical purposes to assess individual children and may not be appropriate for the design of interventions in developing countries.

4. A comprehensive overview of risk factors for child development can be found in the Bright Futures guidelines (Council on Children with Disabilities, 2006). In this document, risk factors are grouped on the basis of the transactional model, i.e. risks related to the child, family and community. Again, while this framework may be useful at an individual level, health systems in developing countries may find it difficult to use, as programmes are not usually structured in this way. Neither the DC 0-3 R nor the Bright Futures guidelines consider conditions that are specifically important in LAMI countries, or provide a framework for addressing these conditions.

The life cycle approach to developmental risk factors

We present here a novel conceptual framework for developmental risk factors, which can be used to guide the efforts of LAMI countries to prevent and manage developmental difficulties. The life cycle approach provides a mapping of risk factors in chronological order, from before conception to adulthood, parenthood and the next generation. This approach is analogous with – but more comprehensive than – the approach used in the WHO document, *Mental retardation: from knowledge to action* (WHO, 2006b).

The life cycle approach embodies four key concepts:

1. Risk and protective factors coexist throughout the lifespan, respectively impairing or helping children to develop to their full potential.

2. Factors that place children's survival at risk are also often risks for suboptimal development.

3. Often risks do not occur in isolation but together. The cumulative number, duration and severity of risk factors, and the adequacy of protective factors, determine the ultimate impact of risk factors.

4. Risks affect development through multiple complex pathways, and categorizations, such as biological and psychosocial, or nutritional, genetic and infectious, have limited use. Interventions to address risks must be informed by the multifaceted complex nature of risk and protective factors.

The life-cycle approach comprises the backbone for conceptualization of the prevention of developmental difficulties, as outlined in Chapter 5.

The life-cycle approach is depicted in Figure 2 (Ertem, 2011). In this framework, developmental risks are presented in order of appearance and significance within the life-cycle. There are lifelong risks, which can appear at any time of the life-cycle. These are shown at the centre of the schema and include physical and mental health problems of the caregivers, deficiencies in the psychosocial and educational environment, exposure to substances and toxins, and exposure to vio-

Figure 2. The life-cycle approach to developmental risk factors (reproduced from Ertem, 2011)

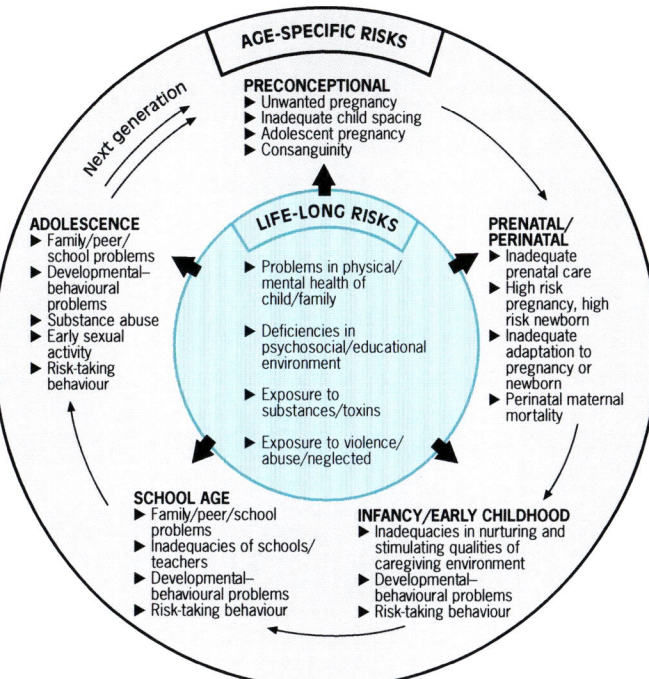

lence, abuse or neglect. There are also age-specific risks, which can appear at specific periods in life: preconception, prenatal/perinatal, infancy/early childhood, school age and adolescence.

Figure 3 shows specific risks that may affect development of children up to the age of 3 years. Deficiencies in the social environment (e.g. in nutrition, housing, environmental hygiene, living-wage jobs, gender equality, child care and school facilities) and physical and mental health problems of the caregiver can affect child development from before conception into the early years of life and beyond. Preventive efforts should be targeted to the entire lifespan. Time-specific risk factors are listed in Figure 3 according to the period during which they can be targeted. For example in order to prevent the negative effects of consanguinity between parents, interventions must be made before conception.

Summary of research from LAMI countries

Resilience and protective factors in young children

There is a need for research on the concept of resilience and developmental protective factors in LAMI countries. One exemplary study of resilience has been carried out in a rural community in India. This study examined the effects of maternal child-rearing behaviour, parental attributes, and socioeconomic status and their association with "positive deviance" in the development of preschool children (Aruna, Vazir & Vidyasagar, 2001). Children whose mothers were responsive to their needs, consistent in their interactions

Figure 3. Specific risks that can affect children up to 3 years of age

Preconceptional	Prenatal/perinatal	Newborn	First years of life
Problems/ deficiencies in maternal health and nutrition	Maternal mortality	Inadequate caregiver–newborn relationship and interactions	Lack of appropriate child care
Inadequate child spacing	Perinatal asphyxia	Neonatal infections, complications	Child health problems/ chronic illness
Unwanted pregnancy	Low birth weight	Developmental/sensory impairments	Inadequacies in nurturing and stimulating qualities of the environment Iron deficiency
Parental consanguinity	Prematurity		Iodine deficiency
	Perinatal complications, infections		Malnutrition
	Congenital chromosomal abnormalities		Micronutrient deficiencies

Exposure to environmental toxins
Problems in caregiver physical and mental health
Deficiencies in the social and economic environment: nutrition, housing, environmental hygiene, living-wage jobs, gender equality, caregiver education, child care, preschool opportunities, schools, access to public and private goods and services, health care, exposure to violence/war.

with them and emotionally stable during specific situations were found to be "positive deviant" (resilient) in their development. Other factors that were significantly associated with positive deviance were paternal literacy and a nuclear family.

Risk factors in young children

There has been a much larger volume of research in developing countries on developmental risk factors. This research is presented here in the life-cycle framework.

1. The preconceptional period

This period spans the life of the parents before the conception of the child. The transition from adolescence to adulthood for both prospective parents is a critical period. Factors detrimental to the physical and mental health of the parents and their parenting role are potential risk factors for early childhood development. It is difficult to study the effect on child development of risks during this period alone because these risks often continue during the prenatal and postnatal period. The challenges related to this period, specifically for young people living in developing countries, have been reviewed by the US National Research Council (Lloyd, 2005).

Social determinants of health and maternal physical and mental health are risk factors that have been reviewed elsewhere; they are therefore not discussed in detail here. There have, however, been no reviews of the literature on parental consanguinity, adolescent parenting, unintended pregnancy and child spacing with particular emphasis on developing countries; research on these risk factors is therefore covered in more detail below.

(a) Social determinants of health. A thorough review of the effects on child development of the social determinants of health was commissioned by WHO (Irwin, Siddiqi & Hertzman, 2007). This document summarized the evidence for the effects on child development of social determinants, such as poverty and low maternal education. It explored the role of risk factors that start before conception and continue across the lifespan. Factors close to the child, including quality of parenting skills, early stimulation and the detrimental effects of being orphaned, as well as factors that are more distant, such as gender-based discrimination; alcohol and substance abuse in the family, dwelling conditions, forced labour, war and famine, are also considered.

(b) Maternal physical health. A recent review for WHO (Hutton, 2006) highlighted the extent to which maternal and newborn ill-health generate additional risks for individuals and families and the role that this plays in the vicious cycle of underdevelopment and poverty.

(c) Caregiver mental health. There is convincing and growing evidence that caregiver mental health problems, in particular depression, that are related to developmental difficulties in children often begin before conception and continue during the early years. Readers are referred to seminal research by Rahman and Patel related to the effects of maternal mental health on child health and development (Patel, DeSouza & Rodrigues, 2003; Patel & Prince, 2006; Patel, 2007; Rahman et al., 2004a, 2004b, 2007, 2008) as well as two recent Lancet series on mental health (Bhugra & Minas, 2007; Barret, 2007; Dhanda, 2007; Herrman & Swartz, 2007; Horton, 2007; Katonka, 2007; Miller, 2007; Sartorius, 2007) and early childhood development (Walker et al., 2007).

(d) Parental consanguinity. In many parts of the developing world, marriages between close biological kin are preferred and may account for 50% of all marriages in certain populations (www.consang.net). Scientific evidence for the effect of consanguinity on children's cognitive development dates back to the 1970s (Bashi, 1977). Offspring of consanguineous parents are over-represented among individuals with neurodegenerative disorders (Ozand, Devol & Generoso, 1992), inborn errors of metabolism (Kabiri, 1982; Ozguc et al., 1993), congenital hypothyroidism (Hashemipour et al., 2007; Karamizadeh & Amrihakimi, 1992), severe mental retardation (Afzal, 1988; Bashi, 1977; Hafez et al., 1985), blindness (Elder & De Cock, 1993), and hearing impairment (Ben Arab, Bonaiti-Pellie & Belkahia, 1990; Kabarity et al., 1981).

Studies from around the world have shown a significantly higher incidence of major congenital malformations in offspring of consanguineous parents (Freire-Maia & Elisbao, 1984; Jaber et al., 1992; Khrouf et al., 1986). Most of the research on consanguinity comes from developing countries, and epidemiological information on consanguineous marriage and its outcomes is sparse, unavailable or inadequate. In a study of 1000 pregnant women in Pondicherry, India, 31% were in a consanguineous marriage, with a higher frequency among those from rural areas and Hindus (Verma, Prema & Puri, 1992). This study reported significantly higher infant mortality and fetal death in consanguineous marriages. On the other hand, surveys in Saudi Arabia (Swailem et al., 1988) and Pakistan (Yaqoob et al., 1993) were unable to detect significantly higher rates of mortality or birth defects. It is important to recognize that, in most countries where consanguineous marriages are common, epidemiological studies are difficult to conduct, congenital disorders may not be correctly diagnosed, and differentiation between genetic and non-genetic determinants of morbidity may be overlooked.

Studies in developed countries have found direct associations between parental consanguinity and childhood developmental difficulties. In Pakistani immigrants in the United Kingdom, 50–55% of marriages are between first cousins (Darr & Modell, 1988). The perinatal mortality in this community in 1988 (15.7 per 1000 births) significantly exceeded that in all other population groups of the United Kingdom, and was consistent across all socioeconomic classes. Congenital anomalies accounted for 41% of all infant deaths among British Pakistanis during the period 1982–85. In another multi-ethnic prospective study, serious malformations were diagnosed in 28.2 per 1000 British-Pakistani babies. Chronic disorders, many with a recessive mode of inheritance, were diagnosed in 41.5 per 1000 of those surviving the first month of life (Bundey & Alam, 1993; Chitty & Winter, 1989).

More recent studies from the United Kingdom draw attention to the continued relationship between developmental difficulties and consanguinity. A study in the northern English city of Bradford showed a relationship between severe disorders, including neurodegenerative disorders, microcephaly and cerebral palsy, and Pakistani immigrants with consanguinity (Corry, 2002). In a study in southern Derbyshire, Pakistani children were found to have a higher prevalence of severe learning disorder, profound hearing loss, severe visual problems, autism and cerebral palsy, and higher disability scores than other groups (Morton et al., 2002). Genetic disease causing disability was ten times more common in Pakistani children than other immigrant groups. Studies on Arab populations in Israel have found an association between parental consanguinity and congenital malformations (Bromiker et al., 2004) and childhood reading disability (Abu Rabia & Maroun, 2005).

It is possible to prevent morbidity related to consanguineous marriages. Research on thalassaemia control in Cyprus (Angastiniotis & Hadjiminas, 1981; Kuliev, 1986) for example, shed light on interventions related to premarital genetic counseling that can be targeted to address consanguineous marriages, with subsequent reduction of recessively inherited disorders in the population. Current evidence points to the need to inform populations about the risk of consanguineous parenting for child development.

(e) Adolescent parenting. Adolescent parenting is an important risk factor for the survival, health and development of both children and their mothers in all countries. A review of the effects of adolescent parenting on maternal and child health, with particular attention to LAMI countries, has been produced by WHO (Treffers, 2002). Another WHO document (Khan, 2004) reviewed the major factors affecting pregnancy outcome among adolecents, socioeconomic barriers to adolescent health care and programmes that have been effective in improving pregnancy outcome. A more recent WHO publication on adolescent pregnancy aims to draw the attention of policy makers and programme managers to the need to improve care for pregnant adolescents, both inside and outside the health care system (McIntyre, 2006).

There has been abundant research in developed countries on the specific effects of adolescent parenting on early childhood development. Research in the 1970s and 1980s indicated that children of adolescent parents were at a slightly increased risk of abuse, but sound empirical data for "suboptimal intellectual development" were lacking (Elster, McAnarney & Lamb, 1983; Roosa, Fitzgerald & Carlson, 1982). Later studies identified numerous challenges for adolescent mothers and their children. Adolescent mothers have been found to have high rates of depression (Colletta, 1983; Leadbeater, Bishop & Raver, 1986; McHenry et al., 1990; Wasserman et al., 1990). Children of adolescent mothers are at higher risk of being maltreated (George & Lee, 1997; Haskett, Johnson & Miller, 1994; Siegel et al., 1996; Stier et al., 1993) and of having developmental and behavioural problems (Coley & Chase-Lansdale, 1998; Furstenburg, Brooks-Gunn & Morgan, 1987; Hubbs-Tait et al., 1994; Lyons-Ruth & Block,1996; Miller & Moore, 1990). A review examining the link between adolescent parenting and developmental delays among the offspring outlined a number of possible causes for this association (Borkowski et al., 1992). Most importantly, the mother–child relationship may be impaired, as adolescent mothers are less likely to have the support of a social network, may be unprepared cognitively and emotionally to assume responsibility for child-rearing, and may have had the baby in an attempt to meet their own needs for nurturing. As a result, the parenting style of adolescents may deprive the child of appropriate nurturing and stimulation, which could be detrimental to the child's development. Other adversities associated with adolescent parenting, such as poverty, can also have a negative impact on child development. Furthermore, in LAMI countries, adolescent pregnancy is more frequently associated with preterm and low birth weight infants (McIntyre, 2006), which in turn may be responsible for increased developmental risk for the offspring. In a study in Delhi, India, complications of pregnancy, such as abnormal presentation and prolonged labour, were more common among adolescents. In this study, the rates of miscarriages and stillbirths were reported to be 17.5% and 3.5% among adolescents and adults, respectively (Sharma et al., 2003).

Many adolescent mothers live with their own parents. In a study examining the effects of adolescent parenting in this situation, Black et al. (2002) found that living in a three-generation household did not protect young children from the effects of depression and maltreatment (Black et al., 2002). Children with the fewest behavioural problems were living with their own mother in their own household and had not been maltreated, and their mothers had fewer symptoms of depression.

There has been little research on the effects of adolescent fathering on child development. Studies in the United States have shown that having a child is a major stress factor for teenage males. However, when teenage fathers take part in child-rearing and the mothers have a positive perception of the father's support, the children tend to have better cognitive ability and behaviour than those without such paternal support (Barret & Robinson, 1990).

Most adolescent pregnancies occur in LAMI countries, where they are a leading cause of maternal death (Mayor, 2004). For example, girls in southern Sudan are more likely to die in childbirth than to complete primary school (Moszynski, 2004). Research on the effects of adolescent parenting on the developmental outcome of children in LAMI countries, however, is extremely limited.

In an Inter-American Development Bank Project, Buvinic (1998) reviewed studies from Chile (Buvinic, 1998), Barbados (Russell-Brown, Engle & Townsend, 1992), Guatemala (Engle, 1993; Engle & Smidt, 1996) and Mexico (Rico & Atkin, 1995) to identify the consequences of adolescent childbearing. The findings showed that, among poor mothers, adolescent childbearing was associated with higher maternal fertility, lower monthly earnings, lack of financial support, and grandparents taking responsibility for child care. The nutritional status of the children was investigated 4–10 years after their birth: significantly more first-born children of adolescent mothers had a height-for-age below the norm, compared with children of older mothers. Children of adolescent mothers also had lower scores on a language-development test and their mothers more frequently reported behavioural problems (Buvinic, 1998). These negative findings were true only for adolescent mothers living in poverty.

Most adolescent pregnancies in high-income countries lead to single parenting, whereas adolescent mothers in LAMI countries are often married and have a different social status than those in industrialized countries. The effects of adolescent parenting on child development, therefore, may be different between countries at different levels of development and between impoverished and wealthier populations. Evidence suggests, nevertheless, that adolescent pregnancy is a major risk factor for the survival, health and development of the mother and child.

(f) Unintended pregnancies. Studies of the relationship between pregnancy intention and birth, maternal and child health, and development outcomes have been conducted largely in developed countries. These studies date back to the 1980s, but they are few in number. Three studies used data from the United States National Longitudinal Survey of Youth. The first study involved 1327 children under two years of age and their mothers (Baydar, 1995). Pregnancies that were mistimed or unwanted were associated with lower scores on scales measuring parental provision of opportunity for children's skill development and non-authoritarian parenting style. During the assessments two years later, children were found to have a significantly less positive relationship with their mother. Children born from an unwanted or mistimed pregnancy had higher mean scores for fearfulness and lower scores for positive affect and receptive language than wanted infants.

Joyce, Kaestner & Korenman (2000) analysed the same data set using information on siblings to control for confounding family variables that may affect child outcomes. They found no significant differences in maternal behaviour or child outcomes between mistimed and wanted pregnancies. Unwanted pregnancy, however, was associated with prenatal and postpartum maternal behaviour that adversely affected infant and child health. In the same cohort, infants whose conception was intended by the mother but not the father were also at elevated risk of adverse health events (Korenman, Kaestner & Joyce, 2002).

Mohllajee et al. (2007), in the United States Centers for Disease Control and Prevention, analysed data from the population-based Pregnancy Risk Assessment Monitoring System for 87 087 women who gave birth between 1996 and 1999 in 18 states. When controlled for demographic and behavioural factors, the data showed that women with an unwanted pregnancy had an increased likelihood of preterm delivery and premature rupture of membranes than women with an intended pregnancy. Women who were ambivalent towards their pregnancy had an increased risk of delivering a low birth weight infant.

While most unintended pregnancies occur in developing countries, few studies have addressed the effects of these pregnancies on child health and development. In a study in the Islamic Republic of Iran, unintended pregnancy was found to be a risk factor for antenatal and postpartum depression (Iranfar et al., 2005). The authors called attention to the need for further research on the role of depression in mediating the effects of unintended pregnancy. A study in Egypt found that unintended pregnancy was a barrier to antenatal care but not to child health care (Youssef et al., 2002).

A study in Bolivia examined the impact of maternally and paternally reported pregnancy intention on the prevalence of early childhood stunting. Data were collected from a nationally representative sample of women and men interviewed in the 1998 Bolivian Demographic and Health Survey. The sample was restricted to last-born, singleton children younger than 36 months, for whom complete anthropometric information was available. Children from unwanted and mistimed pregnancies comprised 33% and 21% of the sample, respectively. Approximately 29% of the maternally unwanted children were stunted, compared with 19% of mistimed and 19% of wanted children. Children between 1 and 3 years of age from mistimed and unwanted pregnancies were at approximately 30% greater risk of stunting than children from intended pregnancies. Infants and toddlers reported by both parents as unwanted had an increased risk of being stunted compared with children both of whose parents intended the pregnancy (Shapiro-Mendoza et al., 2005).

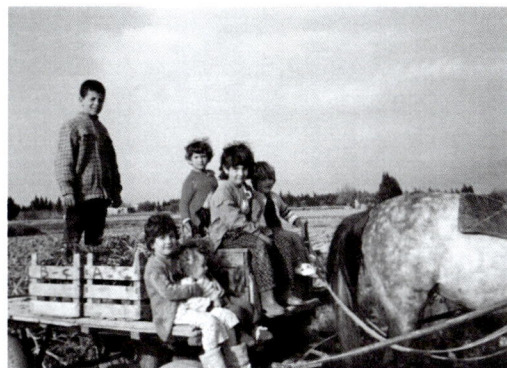

Children develop within the context of their environment: village children, Turkey. Photo: Dr. Cuneyt Ensari

As can be seen from the reviewed literature, there is relatively little evidence for the effects of unintended pregnancy on child development. There is a large amount of information, however, on the association between unintended pregnancy and conditions that are proxy for developmental difficulties in young children, such as malnutrition/stunting, maternal depression, inadequate child spacing, and poverty. Preventing unintended pregnancy, therefore, is likely to be an effective strategy for reducing developmental difficulties in children.

(g) Inadequate birth interval (child spacing). Inadequate birth interval is a well known risk factor for child survival and health. Studies examining the role of birth spacing on child development are relatively new. Hayes et al. (2006) in the United States showed that children born after an inadequate birth interval (less than 24 months) were more likely to fail cognitive skills assessment tests that predict school readiness. This remained true after correcting for various sociodemographic factors.

In a cross-sectional study by Bella & Al-Almaie (2005) in eastern Saudi Arabia, the school performance of children was examined in relation to the length of the interval before and after their birth. Children born after a birth interval longer than 31 months were significantly more likely to score high grades in the year of study and the year before than children born after an interval of less than 17 months. Significantly more children born before a birth interval longer than 35 months did better at school than those born before an interval of less than 19 months. Logistic regression analysis showed that the possibility of classifying the index child's school performance as average or above increased as the succeeding birth interval increased. The study found that the succeeding birth interval was more significant than the preceding birth interval in relation to school performance.

In developing countries, inadequate birth spacing is a risk factor for childhood survival and also indirectly affects child development through its association with increased risk of malnutrition. Rutstein (2005) examined the association between birth interval, infant and child mortality, and nutritional status in a repeated analysis of retrospective survey data from the Demographic and Health Surveys (DHS) in 17 developing countries between 1990 and 1997. For neonatal and infant mortality, the risk of dying decreased with increasing birth interval up to 36 months, after which the risk remained stable. For child mortality, the longer the birth interval, the lower the risk, even for intervals of 48 months or more. There was a pattern of increasing chronic and general undernutrition as birth interval decreased in 14 countries.

Potential implications of such research for LAMI countries include the need to promote optimal birth spacing to improve the likelihood that children will survive, grow well, come to school ready to learn, and continue doing well in school.

2. The prenatal and perinatal period

All of the risk factors that affect the preconceptional period continue to pose risks during the prenatal period. Additionally, maternal ill-health, including obstetric complications, nutritional deficiencies, intrauterine infections and prenatal exposure to toxic substances may affect the development of the central nervous system of the fetus and constitute developmental risks (Committee on Nervous System Disorders in Developing Countries, 2001). Intrauterine growth retardation or low birth weight is an important risk factor that can be prevented by interventions during the preconceptional and prenatal periods. This risk factor, which has a high prevalence in many LAMI countries, has been reviewed in detail in a WHO/UNICEF document (UNICEF, 2004) and in a *Lancet* series (Walker et al., 2007).

Three perinatal risks that have not previously been reviewed in detail in relation to child development in LAMI countries are considered below: prematurity, birth asphyxia and maternal mortality.

a) Prematurity. Widespread application in high-income countries of advances in neonatology over the past few decades has led to the survival of many preterm infants. Numerous studies have been conducted in these countries to follow up premature infants with very low birth weight (VLBW) – defined as birth weight ≤ 1500 g – and more recently of those with extremely low birth weight (ELBW) ≤ 1000 g. Recent reviews of developmental outcome have concluded that premature infants are at increased risk of developmental difficulties (Marlow, 2004). These include major sequelae, such as cerebral palsy (Bhutta et al., 2002; Jongmans et al., 1997; Platt et al., 2007), impaired vision due to retinopathy of prematurity (Quiram & Capone, 2007), and hearing impairment (Ari-Even Roth et al., 2006), as well as difficulties involving cognitive functions, learning and behaviour (Davis et al., 2005a; Hack et al., 1992; Msall & Tremont, 2002; O'Brien et al., 2004; Taylor et al., 1998; Volpe, 1997).

Although the overall survival of preterm infants in LAMI countries is still low, neonatal intensive care technology is advancing rapidly in tertiary health care centres, and many VLBW premature infants that have access to these facilities are surviving beyond the neonatal period (Atasay et al., 2003; Garg & Bolisetty, 2007; Trotman & Barton, 2005).

Over the past decade, a number of studies in LAMI countries have been published on the short-term developmental outcome of premature infants. Examples include: South Africa (Cooper & Sandler, 1997; Kirsten et al., 1995), Malaysia (Boo et al., 1996; Ho et al., 1999), Papua New Guinea (Brown, 1996), China (Province of Taiwan) (Chang et al., 2000), Turkey (Atasay et al., 2003; Özbek et al., 2005), Kenya (Were & Bwibo, 2006) and Bangladesh (Khan et al., 2006). All these studies were single-centre-based, had sample sizes ranging from 25 to 162, and had large rates of attrition in follow-up. Some studies demonstrated developmental morbidity similar to that seen in high-income countries in surviving premature infants (Kirsten et al., 1995; Ho et al., 1999), while others highlighted a higher rate of developmental morbidity (Were & Bwibo, 2006; Chang et al., 2000). In the most recent follow-up studies, in Kenya, at 24 months, 12% of surviving VLBW infants had cerebral palsy, 9% had delayed cognitive skills and 26% had functional disabilities. A follow-up study in Bangladesh of 159 newborns born before 33 weeks gestational age showed that 32% had normal development while 45% had mild and 23% serious neurodevelopmental impairments. Cognitive impairment was the most common deficit (60%) (Khan et al., 2006).

Very few studies have been published on the long-term developmental outcome of premature infants in LAMI countries. The largest cohort was followed by Chaudhari et al. (2000) in Pune, India. Of the 404 high-risk newborns initially enrolled, many with VLBW, 286 were assessed at six years of age. Of these, 14.6% showed borderline intelligence. At 12 years of age, in the VLBW group, 15.4% were intellectually disabled compared with 3.3% in the control group (Chaudhari et al., 2004). Given that attrition was high in the VLBW group, these rates are most likely underestimates. In the cohort of children with birth weight <2000 g assessed at 12 years, parental education and the type of school attended by the child were the most important factors influencing cognitive development. The only biological factor of importance was birth weight, but this made a very small contribution (Chaudhari et al., 2005).

A multisite study from Lebanon reported on 3372 neonates admitted to five National Collaborative Perinatal Neonatal Network Centres. In this study, admissions to the newborn intensive care unit (NICU) were associated with both paternal and maternal education; newborns of illiterate mothers had 3–5 times the risk of NICU admission and prolonged hospitalization (Yunis et al., 2003). This study highlights the fact that social determinants play a crucial role in biomedical risks.

In summary, in comparison with high-income countries, fewer premature or VLBW infants survive in LAMI countries, and a larger proportion have significant developmental difficulties. In both high-income and LAMI countries, higher family income and education mediate resilience in these high-risk children. Efforts to prevent premature birth and to improve the developmental outcome of prematurely born infants are warranted in LAMI countries.

b) **Birth asphyxia.** In a recent review, Azra Haider & Bhutta (2000) drew attention to the public health problem of birth asphyxia in LAMI countries. Birth asphyxia is responsible for approximately 23% of all newborn deaths around the world (Lawn, Shibuya & Stein, 2005). In industrialized countries, improvements in primary and obstetric care have led to a reduction in the incidence of newborn death from birth asphyxia to less than 1 per 1000 births (Badawi et al., 1998). In LAMI countries, rates of birth asphyxia are much higher, ranging from 4.6 per 1000 in Cape Town (Hall, Smith & Smith, 1996) to 26 per 1000 in Nigeria (Kinoti, 1993); case–fatality rates may be 40% or higher (Bang & Bang, 1992). The effects of birth asphyxia on the newborn range from none to severe organ failure and death. According to WHO, between four and nine million newborns experience birth asphyxia each year. Of these, an estimated 1.2 million die and at least the same number develop severe consequences, such as epilepsy, cerebral palsy, and developmental delay (Save the Children, 2001). The numbers of disability-adjusted life years (DALYs) lost due to birth asphyxia estimated by WHO exceed those due to all childhood conditions preventable by immunization (WHO, 2003). However, because community-based data on disability in LAMI countries are rare and there are very few studies reliably assessing the cause of disability, the impact of birth asphyxia on childhood and later adult disability is uncertain.

> In comparison with high-income countries, fewer premature or VLBW infants survive in LAMI countries, and a larger proportion have significant developmental difficulties. In both high-income and LAMI countries, higher family income and education mediate resilience in these high-risk children.

c) **Maternal mortality.** Maternal mortality is defined by WHO as "the death of a woman while pregnant or within 42 days of termination of pregnancy, irrespective of the duration and site of the pregnancy, from any cause related to or aggravated by the pregnancy or its management, but not from accidental or incidental causes". Maternal mortality continues to be the major cause of death among women of reproductive age in many countries. Yearly, 0.36 million maternal deaths occur globally (Nyamtema et al., 2011). Maternal death is well known to be associated with increased neonatal, infant and childhood mortality (Anderson et al., 2007; Rajaram, 1990; Reyes Frausto et al., 1998). Yet, there has been surprisingly little research on the effects of maternal death on later child development, with the exception of death from HIV/AIDS.

A study in Mexico examined the effects of maternal death on family dynamics and infant survival. Family members were interviewed at the time of the death and a year later. The main consequences were found to be family disintegration, children in the family acquiring caregiving and income-generating roles, and economic problems. Children were often integrated in the grandparents' family (Reyes Frausto et al., 1998). The high rates of preventable maternal mortality in LAMI countries must be viewed as a major risk factor affecting child survival, health and early development.

3. Neonatal period.

The concept of the "high-risk newborn" is long-standing and refers to newborn infants that are at high risk for mortality and developmental morbidity. There has been abundant research in developed countries on neonatal risk factors that affect child development, such as hyperbilirubinaemia, hypoglycaemia, sepsis, intracranial infections, and cardiac and pulmonary problems. A comprehensive and practical review of this research has been prepared by Bear (2004).

In LAMI countries, most risk factors that have an impact on neonatal survival also have a potential impact on later development. Readers are referred to the *Lancet* series on neonatal survival (Darmstadt et al., 2005; Lawn et al., 2005; Martines et al., 2005). WHO has produced a useful guide to the management of neonatal complications that are common in LAMI countries (WHO, 1998a).

4. First three years of life.

A number of important documents have been produced containing information on developmental risk factors that need to be addressed during the early years:

- *A critical link* reviews the link between malnutrition and lack of psychosocial stimulation (WHO, 1999).

- *The importance of caregiver-child interactions for the survival and healthy development of young children* provides a comprehensive review of the role of caregiving in child health and development (Richter, 2004).

- *Early childhood development: A powerful equalizer* reviews the social determinants of child development (Irwin, Siddiqi & Hertzman, 2007).

- On its web site, UNICEF provides a list of reviews related to the impact of HIV/AIDS on the development of young children in South Africa (**http://www.unicef.org/southafrica/resources_2805.html**).

- The *Lancet* series on "Early childhood development in developing countries" reviewed risk factors that: (a) can be addressed by interventions or public policy; (b) affect children from before birth up to 5 years of age; and (c) affect large numbers of young children in developing countries (Walker et al., 2007).

  — The biological risks reviewed were: intrauterine growth retardation, undernutrition, iodine deficiency, iron deficiency, breastfeeding and zinc, infectious diseases, and environmental exposure (including to lead, arsenic, manganese and methylmercury, and prenatal pesticide exposure,).

  — The psychosocial risks included were: cognitive stimulation and child learning opportunities, caregiver sensitivity and responsiveness, maternal depression, and exposure to violence.

- The relationship between mental health and child health and development has been addressed in the recent *Lancet* series on mental health (Bhugra & Minas, 2007; Barret, 2007; Chisholm et al., 2007; Dhanda, 2007; Herrman & Swartz, 2007; Horton, 2007; Jacob et al., 2007; Patel et al., 2007; Prince et al., 2007; Saraceno et al., 2007; Sartorius, 2007; Saxena et al., 2007).

The above documents and their references provide a comprehensive overview of individual risk factors that play a role in early childhood development. In this review, particular emphasis will be given to research from LAMI countries that has examined the role of multiple, co-occurring risk and protective factors that affect the development of young children.

(a) Risks associated with emotional and social development and behavioural problems. Three studies in LAMI countries (Brazil, India and the United Arab Emirates) have demonstrated the links between biopsychosocial risk factors and emotional and social development.

In an epidemiological study of 634 preschool children followed from birth in Brazil, the prevalence of behavioural problems was 24%. Maternal psychiatric disorder, education, age, number of younger siblings and quality of the home environment explained 28% of the variance in behavioural problems (Anselmi et al., 2004).

In rural India, a study involving 3746 children

aged less than 6 years examined the environmental factors influencing development. Significant independent factors influencing psychosocial development were: per capita income, education of the mother, nutritional status of the child, number of rooms and environmental hygiene in the home, presence of a high school within easy travel distance, availability of a caretaker when the mother was busy, child attending an anganwadi nursery which is an early childhood setting run by community workers, household access to newspapers, child having toys or toy substitutes, television, books, and story-telling by the mother (Kumar et al., 1997).

Risk factors associated with behavioural problems in 2–3-year-old children in the United Arab Emirates were reported to be perinatal factors, adverse family factors and a history of mental health problems in the family (Eapen, Zoubeidi & Yunis, 2004).

(b) Risks associated with cognitive development. Four studies in LAMI countries (Argentina, Brazil, India and Pakistan) exemplify the evidence for multiple risk and protective factors affecting cognitive development.

In a population-based study in Argentina, Lejarraga et al. (2002) found that, even for healthy low-risk young children, high social class and maternal education were associated with earlier attainment of selected developmental milestones.

In a cohort study in a low-income population in north-eastern Brazil, social factors, most importantly poverty, had a detrimental effect on the cognitive and motor development of 12-month-old children (Lima et al., 2004). In this study, a cohort of 245 infants born in 1998 was followed longitudinally. At 12 months, psychosocial and biological factors associated with Bayley scale scores were examined. Biological factors (birth weight, weight for age, haemoglobin concentration and sex of the infant) explained only 6–8% of the variance in developmental scores, whereas 20% of the variance was explained by poverty-related risk factors (Lima et al., 2004).

The effects of nutrition and home environment on behavioural development and intelligence were examined in 196 children in rural India. Malnourished children scored poorly in all the areas of development (motor, adaptive, language and personal social). Approximately 27% of children with malnutrition had an IQ score less than 79. Maternal involvement and stimulation were strongly associated with better behavioural development and intelligence. Multiple regression analysis showed that the effect of the home environment on development and intelligence was greater than that of social status, family variables and nutritional status (Agarwal et al., 1992).

In Pakistan, young children in lower socioeconomic groups showed delayed development in comparison with their upper middle class counterparts (Yaqoob et al., 1993). In a cross-sectional study of 2000 apparently healthy children aged under 6 years living in urban and rural areas of Jabalpur, higher income emerged as the only real protective factor against poor cognitive development (Dixit, Govil & Patel, 1992).

(c) Risk factors associated with developmental disability. Seven studies from LAMI countries (Afghanistan, Bangladesh, India, Israel, Nigeria, Pakistan and Saudi Arabia) have provided information on risk factors associated with developmental disabilities. One of the earliest such studies was in Nigeria (Izuora, 1985), and examined the causes of mental retardation in a hospital-based sample of 291 children. The high proportion of cases due to birth trauma (23%) or severe neonatal jaundice (9%) reflected inadequacies in the quality of maternal and child services and obstetric care.

In a study on the frequency of mental retardation, screening and diagnostic assessments were carried out in eight developing countries. Approximately 1000 children aged 3–9 years were surveyed in each location. Patterns of risk factors related to mild and severe mental retardation were examined. Parental consanguinity and multiple impairments were found in children with severe mental retardation. Families of children with any degree of mental retardation were found to be of lower socioeconomic status than comparison families of children with no mental retardation (Stein, Belmont & Durkin, 1987).

In a study of chronic conditions and illnesses causing disability in Jewish Israeli children aged 2–3 years, 76 principal medical conditions causing disability were defined. Very low birth weight and family problems were considered the major risk factors for developmental delay or disability. The disability rate among children with these risks was 6–7.5 times greater than in the total population. The most common developmental difficulties were speech and language disorders and undefined developmental delay. These conditions were more prevalent among children of mothers with a low educational level (Palti, Bendel & Ornoy, 1992).

A study in Pakistan found that, in children with

intellectual impairments with onset during the perinatal period (22% of cases), the main underlying risk factors were being small for gestational age and inherited disorders. During the postnatal period (28% of cases), social deprivation and malnutrition were the major causes of intellectual disability. In a substantial proportion of the cases (50%), the onset or cause of intellectual disability could not be traced. This study indicated a clear relationship between mild intellectual disability and prenatal and postnatal malnutrition and social deprivation. Maternal illiteracy and small head circumference at birth were the two variables that showed a clear association with the development of mild mental disability (Yaqoob et al., 2004).

A study on the prevalence of childhood disability in urban India suggested that comparatively small differences in social status were associated with important differences in health status. Random samples of mothers from the lowest and next-to-lowest socioeconomic classes were interviewed to determine the prevalence of serious disability in children aged 2–9 years. Disability was found to be more common among children of the lowest-class families (17.2%) than those of the next-to-lowest class families (8.4%) (Natale et al., 1992).

Risks of developmental disabilities were studied in a preliminary case–control study in Afghanistan, a low-income country with extremely high rates of maternal illiteracy. Mothers and children attending a primary care clinic in Afghanistan were enrolled. The majority of mothers were illiterate (97%) and only 22% had received antenatal care. The major risk factors for disability were consanguinity (first-cousin parents) and lack of antenatal care. In this study, presentations of disability were found to be: delayed physical and mental development (25% of cases), cerebral palsy (13%), club foot (10%), hearing impairment (9%), and visual impairment (2%) (Nasir et al., 2004). A study in the north-east region of India showed that, of 376 children in a special school, 36% had developed visual impairment as a result of vitamin A deficiency (Bhattacharjee et al., 2008).

In an epidemiological study in Saudi Arabia, early and late marriage and childbearing, as well as low education, unemployment, multiparity and consanguineous marriage, were found to be risk factors contributing to developmental disabilities in children (Shawky, Abalkhail & Soliman, 2002).

Prenatal and postnatal risk factors for mental retardation among children were studied in approximately 10 300 children aged 2–9 years in Bangladesh. Multivariate analysis revealed that prenatal, perinatal, neonatal, and postnatal factors all contributed to the prevalence of cognitive disabilities. Significant independent predictors of serious mental retardation in rural and urban areas included maternal goitre and postnatal brain infection. In rural areas, consanguinity and landlessness were also independently associated with serious mental retardation. In both rural and urban areas, independent risk factors for mild cognitive disabilities included maternal illiteracy, landlessness, maternal history of pregnancy loss, and the child being small for gestational age at birth. The authors suggested that "interventions likely to have the greatest impact on preventing cognitive disabilities among children in Bangladesh include expansion of existing iodine supplementation, maternal literacy, and poverty alleviation programs as well as prevention of intracranial infections and their consequences" (Durkin et al., 2000).

(d) Lack of appropriate child care. The effects on child development of lack of appropriate care have been well investigated in high-income countries. In such countries, most young children and their families have access to high-quality child care and preschool settings, and leaving a child at home alone is considered neglect or abuse. Children in LAMI countries, who do not have access to other adult caregivers when the primary carer is working or not available, may be left alone or in the care of other children. The scope of the problem is alarming and is only now being investigated. Heymann (2006) produced a groundbreaking study devoted to understanding how globalization is affecting working families around the world. This study reported new findings from an analysis of surveys of 55 000 people from around the world, with over 1000 in-depth interviews of families and policy data from over 160 countries. The report describes how lack of support for working families not only dramatically affects the world's children but also exacerbates gender and income inequalities. An estimated 930 million children under 15 years are being raised in households where all of the adults work, and 36%

> An estimated 930 million children under 15 years are being raised in households where all of the adults work, and 36% of the families interviewed had left a young child at home alone. A further 27% had left a child in the care of another – paid or unpaid – child.

of the families interviewed had left a young child at home alone. A further 27% had left a child in the care of another – paid or unpaid – child. Of parents with an income under US$ 10 per day, 67% have had to choose between losing pay and leaving sick children at home alone. In 66% of the families, where parents had to leave children at home alone or with a child, the children had suffered accidents or other emergencies. In 35% of the cases, the children were reported to have suffered from developmental or behavioural problems. Heymann's work shows the acute consequences of the lack of appropriate child care, particularly in developing countries, but also in more affluent countries without appropriate child care policies. Interventions are urgently needed to combat the chronic effects of being left alone and of lack of appropriate care in the first three years of life.

5. Risks and protective factors across the lifespan

The early years are important for brain development and plasticity, but are not the end-point. There is evidence from longitudinal studies in developed countries that early intervention with at-risk populations is effective, but that the long-term results are also affected by children's experiences in later years. Research related to the Infant Health and Development Program (1990), the Brooklyn Early Education Project (Pierson, 1974), the Abecedarian Project (Campbell et al., 2002), and the Parent-Nurse Partnership Program (Olds et al., 2007) has provided important information on risks, protective factors and the role of interventions across the lifespan. Efforts to address risk factors in the early years should be coupled with efforts to address other risk factors as children grow and mature into school age, adolescence and early adulthood.

Conclusions and implications for action

1. The prevention, early recognition and management of developmental difficulties in young children cannot be accomplished without information on risk factors that adversely affect child development and protective factors that promote child development in adverse circumstances. A life-cycle approach to developmental risk factors is proposed as a guide for the health system to interventions that can reduce risks and increase protective factors.

2. There are many risk factors in developing countries that have an impact on child development. Risk factors often have both biological and psychosocial pathways, and act cumulatively. Most of these risk factors (e.g. maternal illiteracy, malnutrition, intrauterine growth retardation, consanguinity between parents, adolescent pregnancy, lack of pre- and perinatal health care, poor child spacing, unintended pregnancy) are preventable and have been or are being addressed in affluent countries.

3. The identification of risk factors is not only important for the prevention of developmental difficulties, but also for the prevention of conditions that contribute to the severity of developmental disabilities (such as malnutrition).

4. In the life-cycle approach, risk factors can be grouped according to when they can be addressed – in the preconceptional, prenatal, perinatal, neonatal and postnatal periods. This approach provides a roadmap for LAMI countries, to review where their policies and programmes stand in addressing these risk factors and what more they may need to do. This approach should be viewed as a dynamic learning process, in which new risk and protective factors and interventions to address them can be added and shared between countries when there is evidence of the effect of such factors on child development.

5. The DDEC Survey indicated that health care providers in LAMI countries in particular do not have adequate knowledge and experience in recognizing developmental risk factors in young children. The role of individual risk factors, their composite effects and prevention and early recognition should be a part of the training of all health care providers.

6. There has been some research from LAMI countries providing evidence for the effects of social risk factors, such as poverty, on child development. However, research on important core risks, such as child spacing, unintended pregnancy, problems in caregiver physical and mental health and caregiver-child relationships, and deficiencies in child care, is inadequate. These known risk and protective factors, as well as other factors that may be unique to particular cultures, will need to be further investigated, to guide interventions to reduce risks and strengthen protective factors to promote optimal child development.

> WHO provides comprehensive guidance on
> counselling families on care: to improve feeding practices
> and interactions with children, respond effectively when a child is
> sick, stimulate growth and development through play
> and communication activities, and solve
> problems in care.
>
> WHO, 2001c

Chapter 5

Prevention of developmental difficulties

DDEC Survey results

Question 6 of the DDEC Survey (see Annex 1) asked what proportion of all children received preventive services and whether they were free of charge, i.e. paid by government or other insurance and free or at minimal cost to families. Antenatal primary health care for pregnant women, delivery by trained birth attendants, primary health care in the first three years of life, growth monitoring, nutritional counselling, iron supplementation to prevent anaemia, iodized salt, basic immunizations, developmental surveillance, counselling of caregivers on how to improve their child's development, and home-visiting by health care providers were free of charge in most countries. Preventive services, such as antenatal screening for Down syndrome and neonatal screening for phenylketonuria, hypothyroidism and hearing loss, were not free of charge in most LAMI countries. Monitoring of developmental delay using standardized instruments was also not free of charge in most countries.

In most of the LAMI countries surveyed, the majority of children did not receive preventive services. While developmental surveillance, counselling and home-visiting were free of charge, these services did not reach more than half of the population in any LAMI country. The services that were not free of charge reached only a small minority of children.

Purpose of chapter and additional key resources

This chapter presents an overview of interventions that can be delivered through the health care system to prevent developmental difficulties in young children. It includes a theoretical framework for interventions within the health system, examples of research on prevention in LAMI countries, and the WHO/UNICEF Care for Child Development intervention, a model that aims to prevent lack of appropriate stimulation during early childhood. Readers are referred to the third paper in the *Lancet* series, "Early childhood development in developing countries" (Engle et al., 2007), which reviewed a range of interventions to promote child development in developing countries. A review of interventions in high-income countries that have been delivered through the health system is also available (Regalado & Halfon, 2001). An entire issue of the *International Journal of Mental Health Promotion* was devoted to the European Early Promotion Project, a preventive intervention that aimed to promote the mental health of young children in five European countries (Davis & Tsiantis, 2005). A comprehensive review of prevention of disability can be found in a recent document prepared for the Ministry of Health of British Columbia, Canada (Kelly, 2007). Other reviews and documents have dealt with: preventive interventions related to neonatal risks (Greenough, Milner & Dimitriou, 2000; Halliday & Ehrenkrantz, 2000; Henderson-Smart et al., 2000; Jobe, 1993; National Institute of Health, 1995); postnatal factors, including nutrition (Grantham-McGregor & Baker-Henningham, 2005; WHO, 1999); micronutrients (Lozoff & Georgieff, 2006); immunizations (www.who.int/topics/poliomyelitis; www.who.int/immunization/topics/tetanus); infectious diseases (Graves & Gelband, 2006; www.who.int.entity/hiv/pub); social inequalities (Irwin, Siddiqi & Hertzman, 2007); and caregiver–child relationships (Richter, 2006; Eshel et al., 2006; WHO 1998b).

Conceptualization

The United Nations Convention on the Rights of the Child calls for all countries to help children develop to their utmost potential (United Nations, 1989). International organizations, such as WHO and UNICEF, recognize that health care systems can no longer focus solely on the survival of children (Engle, Castle & Menon, 1996; Engle et al., 2007; Grantham-McGregor et al., 2007; Hill, Kirkwood & Edmond, 2004; WHO, 1999). To increase the well-being of both children and adults in LAMI countries, and to prevent developmental difficulties, opportunities to promote early development need to be created and used (Herztman & Power, 2004; Richter, 2003; Simeonsson, 2000). There is substantial information from high-income countries on how child development can be promoted through preventive health care services for young children (Brazelton, 1999; Dworkin, 2004; Green, 1994; Hornstein, O'Brien & Stadtler, 1997; Knight et al., 2001; Mc Learn et al., 1998; Minkovitz et al., 2001; Needleman et al., 1991; Puura et al., 2002; Roberts et al., 2002; Weitzman et al., 2004; Zuckerman et al., 1997, 2004a, 2004b). This approach encounters multiple barriers in health care systems in LAMI countries. Financial limitations are by far the most overwhelming; other major barriers include the paucity of simple models for interventions that can reach large populations and of methods to evaluate their efficacy and effectiveness in LAMI countries (Richter, 2003). A systematic and comprehensive conceptualization of how to promote child development and methods to prevent developmental difficulties within the health systems is needed. To meet this need, we present here a model for preventing developmental difficulties in early childhood.

A model for preventing developmental difficulties in early childhood

The model outlined below aims to assist health care policy-makers to visualize the types of interventions that could be instituted within the health care delivery system to prevent suboptimal development in early childhood. It parallels the schema developed by Kerber et al. (2007) for child survival and health, which highlighted the importance of continuity of care, both throughout the life-cycle (adolescence, pregnancy, childbirth, the postnatal period, and childhood) and between places of caregiving (including households, communities, outpatient and outreach services, and

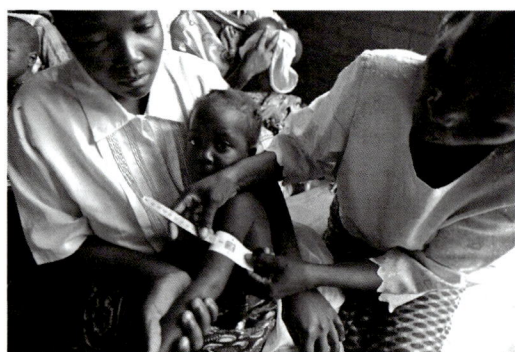

Prevention of malnutrition is crucial to preventing developmental difficulties: health care providers and child, Kenya. © UNICEF/NYHQ2008-1455/Bonn

clinical care settings, such as hospitals). This implies a continuum of interventions, such as reproductive health, obstetric care, antenatal care, postnatal care, care of sick newborn babies and children, child health services, and integrated family and community care, throughout the lifecycle.

The conceptualization of preventive interventions for developmental difficulties is not substantially different from that for child health and survival. The use of similar terminology in the two schemas highlights the significant and striking overlap. The model described here includes the health and survival interventions that prevent developmental difficulties as well as illness and death, and adds others that are directly related to early childhood development, such as enabling caregivers to provide a nurturing and stimulating environment.

The model, shown in Figure 4, has four components, designating when, where and how to intervene and the level of intervention.

1. When to intervene

The timing of an intervention depends on when it will have a preventive effect. The healthy developmental trajectory of a child is influenced throughout the life course by risk and protective factors. Within the life-cycle framework (see page XX), risks and protective factors for developmental difficulties occur at the following times: preconception, prenatal/perinatal, newborn, infancy and early childhood, school age, adolescence and adulthood. In Figure 4, the columns represent the different periods in the life cycle. Interventions are then placed in the column corresponding to the period in which they need to be delivered to prevent developmental difficulties. For example, interventions for improving the social determinants of health can take place throughout the life-cycle, while promotion of adolescent health, prevention of adolescent pregnancy and folic acid and iron supplementation must be carried out before conception.

2. Where to intervene

The places for intervention are represented by the three rows in Figure 4. As proposed by Kerber et al. (2007), family and community care indicates national and community awareness, and support programmes that reach families through media, health providers, educators or other community members. Outpatient and outreach services are delivered through primary health care facilities, and clinical services are health clinic or hospital-based services. For example, while maternal physical and mental health can be promoted at family and community level, early detection and treatment of a problem, such as maternal depression, would be at outpatient or outreach health care level.

3. How to intervene

Interventions for which there is an evidence base, and that have been shown to be deliverable in many countries and to promote child development and prevent difficulties, are listed in Figure 4.

4. Level of intervention

Public health interventions can be at the primary, secondary or tertiary level. The level of each intervention listed in Figure 4 is reflected in the colour of the text.

a) Primary prevention involves preventing the occurrence of disease. A well known example of primary prevention is immunization to prevent illness and disability, e.g. immunization against poliomyelitis. Primary-level interventions for child development include all interventions that aim to prevent risk factors for child development or to promote protective factors that foster resilience. The WHO/UNICEF Care for Child Development intervention is described below as an example of a primary-level intervention. With a life-cycle approach, education of girls, prevention of adolescent pregnancy, promotion of physical and mental health in pregnancy, prevention of birth asphyxia, promotion of safe delivery, prenatal screening, prevention of neonatal infections, malnutrition, iron, iodine and vitamin deficiencies, and promotion of appropriate nurturing and stimulation within the caregiving environment of children are all examples of primary prevention.

b) Secondary prevention involves addressing specific risks after they happen, to prevent the occurrence or reduce the severity of a disease or disorder. A classic example is the early detection and treatment of iron deficiency anaemia. Other examples of secondary prevention efforts are: providing parenting education to high-risk groups, such as adolescents; appropriate risk management for the newborn, such as successful resuscitation and transportation and early recognition and treatment of neonatal jaundice and infections, malnutrition and iron-deficiency anaemia; kangaroo mother care for low birth weight infants; early intervention to promote the development of high-risk infants, such as those with birth asphyxia, low birth weight or prematurity; and early recognition and treatment of maternal depression.

c) Tertiary prevention is defined as specific care, rehabilitation and treatment of conditions when they have occurred, in an effort to prevent further illness or disability. Examples for developmental difficulties are described in detail in Chapter 9.

Using this model, health care providers and policy-makers can determine which interventions need to be delivered to prevent developmental difficulties, when in the life-cycle they need to be delivered, where within systems, and the level of intervention. Although interventions are shown separately on this schema, developmental risks often occur together and affect development through multiple pathways. Similarly, interventions will need to occur in conjunction or along a continuum, to produce a cumulative effect.

Research in LAMI countries

While successful results have been reported for interventions to prevent developmental difficulties in young children (Cooper et al., 2002; Grantham-McGregor, Schofield & Harris, 1983; Grantham-McGregor, Schofield & Powell, 1987; Grantham-McGregor et al., 1991; Hill, Kirkwood & Edmond, 2004; Powell et al., 1995; Super, Herrera & Mora, 1990; WHO, 1999), LAMI countries are still not benefiting from the latest knowledge (Richter, 2003). In reponse to the growth of information on the importance of the early years, and the determinants of health and development across the lifespan (Dawson, Ashman & Carver, 2000; DiPietro, 2000; Hertzman & Power, 2004; Shonkoff & Phillips, 2001), developed countries have been redefining primary care for the past

Figure 4. Model for preventing developmental difficulties in early childhood

	Preconception	Prenatal/perinatal	Newborn	First years of life
CLINICAL CARE		Emergency obstetric care and immediate emergency care for newborn babies Skilled obstetric care at birth and essential care for neonates (hygiene, warmth, breastfeeding)	Appropriate tertiary care for high-risk newborn Extra care for low birth weight newborns, including kangaroo mother care	Emergency care and intensive care Management of childhood illnesses and disorders
OUTPATIENT AND OUTREACH SERVICES	Folic acid and iron supplementation Family planning Genetic screening and counselling	Referral of high-risk pregnancies to tertiary centres Antenatal corticosteroids Termination of pregnancy for detected abnormalities Tetanus immunization Prevention of prenatal infections Prenatal screening Pregnancy follow-up Elective abortion for unintended pregnancies	Extra visits for low birth weight newborns Early recognition and treatment of neonatal jaundice and infections Early detection and referral of neonatal complications Newborn screening	**Community-based rehabilitation** **Early intervention for children with developmental difficulties** **Early detection and management of developmental difficulties** *Early intervention for children at risk of developmental difficulties* *Early detection and treatment of iron deficiency* *Parenting education for high-risk groups (e.g. adolescents)* Developmental and behavioural monitoring and support Prophylactic iron supplements Promotion of caregiver knowledge and skills to provide nurturing and stimulating environment for young children Health supervision visits Home visiting Vaccinations Nutritional counselling and growth monitoring
		INTEGRATED MANAGEMENT OF CHILDHOOD ILLNESSES		
		EARLY DETECTION AND TREATMENT OF MATERNAL DEPRESSION		
FAMILY AND COMMUNITY	Prevention of adolescent pregnancy Reproductive health Adolescent health Education of girls	Recognition of danger signs, emergency preparedness Counselling and preparation for newborn care Preparation for parenthood Reduction of workload	Promotion of mother–newborn and family bonding Prevention of neonatal infections Exclusive breastfeeding	Prevention of violence, abuse and neglect Early recognition and caregiver management of diarrhoea with oral rehydration salts Salt iodinization Promotion of parenting competence for optimal development

PROMOTION OF CHILD, FAMILY AND COMMUNITY RESILIENCE →

PROMOTION OF MATERNAL PHYSICAL AND MENTAL HEALTH →

IMPROVEMENT OF SOCIAL DETERMINANTS OF HEALTH – healthy nutrition, safe housing, environmental hygiene, living-wage jobs, gender equality, appropriate child care, preschool opportunities and schools, access to public and private goods and services, access to health care and appropriately trained health care providers.

Primary prevention; *Secondary prevention*; **Tertiary prevention**

25 years. As a result, in such countries primary health care now addresses a broad range of psychosocial and developmental issues (Black, 2002; Chamberlin, Szumowski & Zastowny, 1979; Chamberlin & Szumowski, 1980; Dinkevich & Ozuah, 2002; Dworkin, 2004; Glascoe et al., 1998; Haggman-Laitila, 2003; Halfon et al., 2004; Puura et al., 2002; Regalado & Halfon, 2001; Schor & Elfenbein, 2004; Thomasgard & Metz, 2004). In LAMI countries, however, structures and concepts such as well-child care, continuity of care, anticipatory guidance, prevention and early identification of developmental delay, and early intervention are still not well established.

We give here a brief summary of findings from research that has not previously been reviewed, categorized according to the level of prevention.

1. Primary prevention.

There are many models of primary prevention from high-income countries. In the United States, for example, children from low-income families are referred to Early Head Start Programs, which provide a range of interventions to improve health, nutitional status, parental competence, and child development (McAllister et al., 2005). In the United Kingdom, Sure Start is a nationwide preventive programme for young children (Roberts & Hall, 2000). Research in developed populations has shown that promotion of development during paediatric health care encounters has many potential benefits for children and families (Davis & Tsiantis, 2005; Margolis et al., 2001; Regalado & Halfon, 2001; Whitt & Casey, 1982). Notwithstanding the increasing popularity of such models, the efficacy of including a child development intervention in a health care encounter has not been fully investigated (Regalado & Halfon, 2001). The limited number of studies has been attributed to the novelty of the field and the difficulty of conducting trials to test efficacy and effectiveness (Zuckerman, Augustyn & Parker, 2001).

In LAMI countries, research on interventions specifically aimed at preventing developmental difficulties is extremely rare.

Three studies are described here as examples of postnatal primary prevention interventions. The first study was on the home-based maternal record (HBMR), which is a practical tool that integrates a number of primary health care interventions, such as prenatal care, immunizations, growth and nutrition. The HBMR allows caregivers and health providers to keep track of a mother and child's health needs and progress. The HBMR is also a system for recording risk factors and early signs of complications, referrals, and treatment of the mother and infant. Data are entered in the record by a number of people, including the mother and various health care personnel. This record also has the potential to address development, and many countries have informal HBMRs that include information on child development as well as child health. The initial WHO HBMR was developed in 1982. A collaborative study in 1984–88 in eight countries (Egypt, India, Pakistan, Philippines, Senegal, Sri Lanka, Yemen and Zambia) to evaluate use of the record summarized its findings as follows: "use of the HBMR had a favourable impact on utilization of health care services and continuity of the health care of women during their reproductive period. The HBMR succeeded in promoting self-care by mothers and their families and in enhancing the timely identification of at-risk cases that needed referral and special care. The introduction of the HBMR increased the diagnosis and referral of at-risk pregnant women and newborn infants, improved family planning and health education, led to an increase in tetanus toxoid immunization, and provided a means of collecting health information in the community. The HBMR was liked by mothers, community health workers and other health care personnel because, by using it, the mothers became more involved in looking after their own health and that of their babies. Apart from local adaptation of the HBMR, the training and involvement of health personnel (including those at the second and tertiary levels), from the start of the HBMR scheme, influenced its success in promoting maternal and child health care. The HBMR also improved the collection of community-based data and the linking of referral networks." (Shah et al., 1993).

The second study, in Brazil, showed the effectiveness of a short-term, primary preventive intervention for child development. In this controlled study on 156 children, those in the intervention group took part in home-based individual and community-based group activities. Two occupational therapists, specialized in child development, and five home visitors delivered the intervention, which comprised of 14 contacts – an initial home visit when the child was 13 months of age, three workshops, and ten reinforcement home visits. At the first home visit, the trainers reviewed the importance of early childhood development and provided examples of appropriate activities for the children. The workshops, which were held when the child was 14, 15, and 16 months of age, included eight mothers in each group and lasted three hours. The 15-month workshop focused on letting the mothers play and interact with their child. Manufactured toys were used during the first part of the session; then the same activity was demonstrated with a home-made toy. For example, a drum was replaced by a tin and spoon, and a shaker by a clear plastic bottle containing coloured bottle tops. Mothers practised making toys from discarded household items and using them to promote specific aspects of development. They also learned how to use everyday activities (e.g. bathing and dressing the child) and everyday household tasks (e.g. laundry and meal preparation) to promote interaction and development. At the 16-month workshop, mothers were encouraged to talk about what they had learned; each group made a poster to illustrate their knowledge of child development and their opinions about the intervention activities. Ten weekly home visits occurred when the child was between 14 and 18 months, as reinforcers. These lasted 30–45 minutes, during which the visitor and mother played with the child in ways that would promote development. At each visit, the visitor left with the mother a toy made from recycled material. The control grouped received regular care at the health fascilities and no intervention. At 18 months, the mean differences between the intervention and control groups were + 9.4 points for Bayley Mental Development Index and + 8.2 points for Psychomotor Development Index ($P < 0.001$ in each case). This study showed the efficacy of a short-term primary intervention to improve the development of young children (Eickmann et al., 2003).

The third study, also in Brazil, showed the effect on mother–child interactions of a one-time intervention (Wendland-Carro, Piccinini & Millar, 1999). First-time mothers were provided with one of two interventions shortly after childbirth: a short videotape and discussion meant to enhance mother–infant interaction, or a control intervention focused on basic caregiving skills. Both interventions were carefully controlled to give the same amount of attention to all mothers. Follow-up at one month showed that the first group was more responsive to, and engaged in more physical contact with, their infants.

2. Secondary prevention

The pioneer for secondary-level prevention research (i.e. addressing specific risks after they happen to prevent the occurrence or reduce the severity of disease) in resource-rich countries was the Infant Health and Development Program (IHDP), conducted in the 1980s in the United States (Brooks-Gunn, Liaw & Klebanov, 1992; Cervantes & Raabe, 1991; Gilette et al., 1991; Kraemer & Fendt, 1990; McCormick et al., 1991; Ramey et al., 1992; Spiker et al., 1991). There has also been considerable research on secondary prevention in LAMI countries.

The WHO publication, *A Critical Link*, reviewed research on many nutritional and psychosocial interventions that address developmental difficulties in children with malnutrition (WHO, 1999). This document also highlighted the importance of applying the biopsychosocial and cumulative risk models in preventive efforts. The work of Grantham-McGregor, who has devoted years to research on secondary-level interventions for malnourished children in Jamaica (Grantham-McGregor et al., 1991), and Bangladesh (Hamadani et al., 2006), provides strong evidence that secondary preventive efforts can be successful.

Secondary interventions can also target caregivers to alter the effect of a risk factor. In South Africa, for example, mother–child interaction was positively affected by 22 intensive, one-hour sessions delivered by trained community health workers to depressed women with young children. The intervention started prenatally and continued until the child was 6 months of age (Cooper et al., 2002).

Examples of other interventions can be found in other reviews (Eshel et al., 2006; Engle et al., 2007).

3. Tertiary prevention

Research in LAMI countries on tertiary prevention for developmental difficulties is reviewed in Chapter 9.

An exemplary model from a developing country: the WHO/UNICEF Care for Child Development Intervention

WHO and UNICEF developed the Care for Child Development Intervention (CCDI) (WHO, 2001c) as a systematic, cost-effective strategy to promote the health and development of young children that can be applied across a variety of public health care settings within resource limitations. The CCDI was initially developed as a supplemet to the Integrated Management of Childhood Illness (IMCI) strategy (Gove, 1997; Lambrechts, Bryce & Orinda, 1999; Pelto et al., 2004; Tulloch, 1999), to promote the development of young children during their encounters with the health care system. There are major differences in the health care delivered to children in high-income and LAMI countries. Children in LAMI countries generally have far fewer encounters with health care providers, and these are typically for acute illness rather than for well-child care. The CCDI makes use of these encounters, and is designed to be used for children with malnutrition, iron deficiency anaemia or an acute minor illness, or for any child under two years who comes into contact with the health care system. Once the reason for the visit has been addressed, the health care provider conducts a standardized semi-structured interview with the primary caregiver, assessing certain aspects of the caregiving environment, specifically how the caregiver plays and communicates with the child. The intervention includes strategies for listening and observing for positive interactions, using specific praise and positive reinforcement, and providing the caregiver with ideas for communication and home-made toys for age-appropriate stimulation.

The CCDI has three important characteristics that make it a promising intervention for worldwide use. First, it is informed by, and reflects, the current "state of the art" teachings on child development. It makes use of caregiver and child competencies in interaction and simple home-made toys for stimulation of child development. Second, the CCDI has been designed for use as a public health intervention in any population, including resource-poor groups in the developing world. In such settings, the only opportunity for health care staff to have contact with caregivers and children may be during consultations for acute illness. Third, the CCDI has a "vector" – the IMCI – so it can be implemented in any country that wishes to take up the IMCI model. Currently many countries that are using the IMCI have expressed an interest in using the CCDI, and some have implemented this intervention within their health systems. WHO and UNICEF are in the process of revising the CCDI so that it can be applied as a "stand-alone" intervention or incorporated into other programmes, such as newborn care and growth monitoring. Research on the CCDI has not been extensive. Pilot studies in Brazil (Dos Santos et al., 1999) and South Africa (Chopra, 2001) suggested that the CCDI could be taught effectively and that the training course improved the knowledge and attitudes of health care providers regarding counselling of caregivers, and could teach health care workers sustained skills that they could then deliver accurately in regular clinical contexts.

In a controlled trial, Ertem et al. (2006) tested the efficacy of the Care for Child Development Intervention in Ankara, Turkey. The study showed

> **The CCDI has three important characteristics that make it a promising intervention for worldwide use. First, it is informed by, and reflects, the current "state of the art" teachings on child development. Second, the CCDI has been designed for use as a public health intervention in any population. Third, the CCDI has a "vector" – the IMCI – so it can be implemented in any country that wishes to take up the IMCI model.**

that the CCDI was safe to use in acute health care visits for children 2 years of age and under, and that the intervention, when reinforced at a second health care visit, was effective in fostering caregivers' efforts to provide a more stimulating home environment for their children. The use of the CCDI can allow child development concepts to be integrated in health care systems in a brief and practical intervention. WHO and UNICEF are further promoting the CCDI as a promising strategy to enhance child development in developing countries.

Conclusions and implications for action

1. The DDEC Survey found that, in most of the countries, many services related to the prevention of developmental difficulties in young children were government-subsidized and

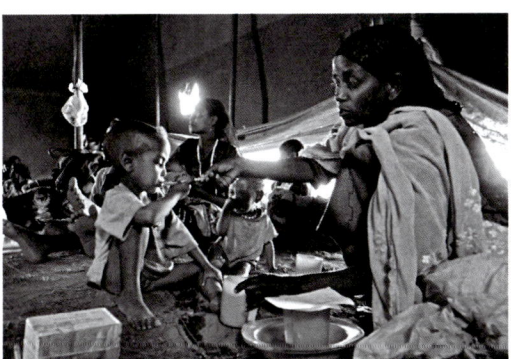

Adequate nutrition is a prerequisite for healthy brain development: children in therapeutic feeding center, Ethiopia. © UNICEF/NYHQ2008-0444/Tegene

free of charge. However, few of these services reached the majority of children, particularly in LAMI countries. Services that were directly related to the prevention of specific disorders, such as neonatal screening, and those related to the promotion of early childhood development, such as counselling caregivers on child development and developmental surveillance, were delivered to very few children in LAMI countries, even though they have been found to be cost-effective in high-income countries.

2. There have been very few studies that have directly examined the effectiveness of interventions to prevent developmental difficulties in young children. Most such interventions are related to nutritional and micronutrient supplementation. There is a great need for studies of effectiveness at all levels of prevention, as well as model programmes in LAMI countries.

3. There is substantial information on how preventive interventions for developmental difficulties can be incorporated into health care for young children in high-income countries. While financial limitations are by far the most overwhelming barrier, the lack of application of knowledge from high-income countries, the paucity of simple models of interventions that can reach mass populations, and the paucity of methods to evaluate their efficacy and effectiveness, are all major impediments to the promotion of preventive interventions in LAMI countries.

4. The framework developed in Chapter 4 can be expanded as a model for viewing preventive interventions. This approach describes primary, secondary and tertiary level interventions that can be applied through the health system. Using this model, countries and communities can visualize what they have already accomplished with regard to preventive interventions and what additional interventions they need to institute to prevent developmental difficulties.

Chapter

Early detection of developmental difficulties

DDEC Survey results

In the DDEC Survey, questions 11 and 14 were specifically related to early detection (see Annex 1). In most countries, caregivers were generally the first to recognize that a young child had developmental difficulties, followed by paediatricians and other health care providers. In most countries, most health providers were not using any instruments routinely to determine the presence of developmental difficulties in young children.

Purpose of chapter

Early recognition of developmental difficulties in young children allows both preventive and therapeutic approaches to be taken and is a crucial step in addressing the problems. In developed countries, the early detection of developmental difficulties is possible because developmental monitoring is an integral part of health care encounters (Baird & Hall, 1985; Blair & Hall, 2006; Council on Children With Disabilities, 2006; Davis & Tsiantis, 2005; Earls & Hay, 2006; Katz et al., 2002; McKay, 2006; Regalado & Halfon 2001; Roberts, 2000; Zuckerman et al., 2004a, 2004b). This chapter promotes "developmental monitoring" as a process for the early detection of developmental difficulties in LAMI countries. It summarizes the conceptualization of early detection and developmental monitoring and addresses key questions that are of importance for LAMI countries in light of the existing research.

Conceptualization

The terms "developmental monitoring", "developmental screening", and "developmental surveillance" have been used interchangeably in the literature. The term "developmental monitoring" is adapted from the definitions of developmental surveillance by Dworkin (1989) and Blair & Hall (2006). The term developmental monitoring is used here for approaches in which a health care provider, who follows the child and family regularly, uses standardized instruments to monitor the child's developmental functioning in all areas. In this model, the child's cognitive, language, social-emotional and motor development is followed on a regular basis, in conjunction with other aspects of the child's health and the family's functioning. Monitoring also includes working with the family to provide special support when needed to ensure the child's optimal development. The term developmental screening is used for approaches in which groups of children are screened to ascertain whether they have developmental delay, by testers who do not necessarily have a continuous relationship with the families or access to health or social information other than that provided by the screening instrument.

The major constituents of developmental monitoring are as follows.

1. The clinician conducting the monitoring should build a relationship with the family.

2. The monitoring process should be family-centred and the family should be an active partner in the monitoring process.

3. The monitoring should be comprehensive, so that multiple aspects of the child's health and development and the family's needs and functioning are taken into consideration, rather than just the results of a screening test.

4. Clinically appropriate, standardized, scientifically reliable and valid instruments should be used.

5. The clinician conducting the monitoring should be knowledgeable about theoretical concepts related to child development.

6. Screening for identifiable and treatable conditions, such as hearing problems, and for meta-

bolic, genetic or other disorders should be an integral part of developmental monitoring.

7. The monitoring process should result in a seamless transition to services that will support the child's development when needed.

Research in high-income countries has shown that children and their caregivers benefit from developmental monitoring during health visits in multiple ways:

1. If the child is developing normally, clinicians can provide reassurance, support parenting competence, and provide anticipatory guidance.

2. If the child has a developmental risk or difficulty, this can be detected early and addressed.

3. In both situations, caregivers can be supported and informed about how to enhance their child's development (Baird & Hall, 1985; Blair & Hall, 2006; Council on Children with Disabilities, 2006; Davis & Tsiantis, 2005; Dworkin, 1989; Earls & Hay 2006; Halfon et al., 2004; McKay, 2006; Regalado & Halfon, 2001; Roberts, 2000; Zuckerman et al., 2004a, 2004b).

At a population level, developmental monitoring can provide information about rates of developmental difficulties, so that interventions can be appropriately targeted, their effect monitored and the need for further interventions determined (Engle et al., 2007; Mung'ala-Odera & Newton, 2007). The use of similar methods in developing countries could potentially lead to better sharing of information between researchers, clinicians and policy-makers and improved allocation of funds, and help decrease the ethically unacceptable gaps between services for young children in different countries.

Research in LAMI countries

Research on developmental monitoring in LAMI countries is examined in relation to six important questions, generated from a review of the literature.

1. Should developmental monitoring be conducted in LAMI countries?

Progress towards monitoring child development in LAMI countries has been impeded by reservations about the availability of interventions and the possibility of increasing the burden on already burdened health care systems. Some

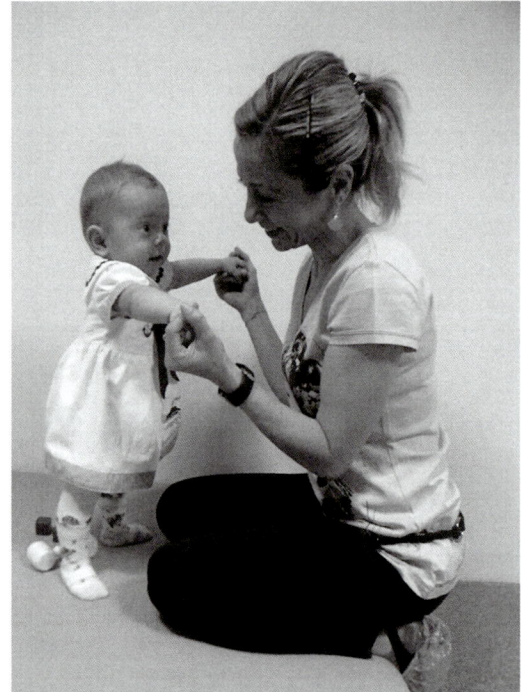

Early detection of developmental difficulties requires active monitoring: child with developmental pediatrician, Turkey. Photo: Dr. Zeynep Eras

authors have suggested that, where services do not exist for children with developmental difficulties, monitoring should not be conducted (Logan, 1995). Although hard data are not available, there is anecdotal evidence that most children with developmental disabilities in LAMI countries do not have access to conventional early intervention and rehabilitation services provided by trained professionals. Even in high-income countries, interventions rely largely on caregivers' involvement with their children during daily activities (Spiker, Hebbeler & Mallik, 2005). Even when professional services are lacking, it is still in the best interest of the child for caregivers to be informed of developmental difficulties and supported in ameliorating development. Furthermore, some developmental difficulties in young children can be treated by a range of interventions that are feasible in many parts of the world, such as nutritional supplementation (Grantham-McGregor & Baker-Henningham, 2005), treatment of iron deficiency (Beard, 2007; Lozoff & Georgieff, 2006; Lozoff, Jimenez & Smith, 2006) improved child–caregiver interaction and infant stimulation (Eshel, 2006; Hamadani et al., 2006; Powell et al., 2004; Richter, 2004; Walker et al., 2005, 2006), and community-based rehabilitation (WHO 2010, Turmusani,Vreede & Wirz, 2002).

Nevertheless, because of this important

reservation, models for developmental monitoring should not be based on a mere screening approach. Such models should incorporate an understanding of risk and protective factors and methods for monitoring and supporting the development of all children within the health care system with direct links to available interventions.

The second reservation – that adding child development concepts may further burden already burdened health care systems – also requires careful consideration. Health care systems in developing countries have conventionally focused on improving child survival rates and physical health. As emphasized in Chapter 2, however, child survival, health and development are closely linked (WHO, 1999). Conditions that have an impact on survival and health, such as malnutrition, also impede development. Conversely, conditions that cause developmental difficulties, such as maternal depression, also have an impact on child survival and health (Klinnert et al., 2001; Rahman et al., 2004a, 2004b, 2007; WHO, 1999). Therefore, models for monitoring child development must be rooted in a child health perspective, and aim to integrate and strengthen efforts to improve child survival and health.

2. **What kinds of instruments are appropriate for developmental monitoring in LAMI countries?**

Instruments that help clinicians to detect developmental difficulties are core components of developmental monitoring, and have evolved in two areas in recent years (Blair & Hall, 2006; Council on Children With Disabilities, 2006; Dworkin, 1989; Gilliam, Meisels & Mayes, 2005; Glascoe, 2005; Meisels & Fenichel, 1996; Meisels& Atkins-Burnet, 2000; Msall, 2005; Rydz et al., 2005). First, language, social-emotional, cognitive and behavioural development and functional capacity have become essential components of instruments. Second, the importance of caregiver–clinician communication and partnership has been reflected in the methods used for developmental monitoring. Based on the family-centred care initiative in child health, illness and advances in early intervention, models in which a parent watches while a clinician "tests" the child have moved to models in which a caregiver and clinician use instruments to "talk" about the child's development and build a joint understanding (Gilliam, Meisels & Mayes, 2005; Glascoe, 2005; Meisels & Fenichel, 1996; Meisels&Atkins-Burnet, 2000). Many instruments that ask caregivers about their concerns regarding their child's development or whether their child has achieved certain developmental milestones have been shown to have appropriate psychometric properties as screening tools and are now recommended in many high-income countries (Council on Children with Disabilities, 2006; Meisels&Atkins-Burnet, 2000). In the USA, the implementation of developmental monitoring and the early detection of developmental difficulties have been effective only when standardized instruments and protocols were used (Bethell et al., 2004; Council on Children with Disabilities, 2006; Meisels&Atkins-Burnet, 2000; Sand et al., 2005; Sices et al., 2004; Zuckerman, 2004b). The American Academy of Pediatrics (AAP), therefore, currently recommends that standardized instruments be used (Council on Children with Disabilities, 2006).

In LAMI countries, the lack of appropriate instruments may be a major barrier to monitoring child development (Engle et al., 2007; Murray & Lopez, 1994; Sonnander, 2000). Studies suggest that caregivers (Ertem et al., 2007; de Lourdes Drachler et al., 2005; Li et al., 2000) and health care providers (Bhatia & Joseph, 2000; Ertem et al., 2007; Figueiras et al., 2003; Kalra, Seth & Sapra, 2005; Lian et al., 2003; Lopez et al., 2000; Mathur et al., 1995; Wirz et al., 2005) in LAMI countries may not have sufficient knowledge about early childhood development and that, therefore, the need for instruments in the monitoring process is even greater than in high-income countries. Some instruments do exist to assess developmental difficulties – for example the "Ten Questions Questionnaire," (Durkin, Hasan & Hasan 1995; Mung'ala-Odera et al., 2004; Thorburn et al., 1992) the "ACCESS portfolio of materials" (Wirz et al., 2005) and the "Disability Screening Schedule" (Chopra, Verma & Seetharaman, 1999; Gupta & Patel, 1991; Mung'ala-Odera & Newton, 2007) do exist. The Ten Questions Questionnaire has proven valuable in many studies in identifying severe disability in older children, but does not aim to provide a framework for monitoring child development. Furthermore, it has been found to be limited in scope (Trani, 2009).

The Denver Developmental Screening Ttest (DDST) (Frankenburg & Dodds, 1967) and the revised version, Denver II (Frankenburg et al., 1992), have been adapted in many countries. This test, however, has the disadvantage of relying on the testing of the child, and requires equipment to elicit a child's skills. It does not provide a description of the child's functioning and does not have a component that can be used for planning interventions. The training does not incorporate the importance of developing partnerships with caregivers. Furthermore, the Denver test has recently lost popularity in the United States as a result of research demonstrating inadequate sensitivity, specificity and accuracy (Glascoe et al., 1992; Glascoe, 2001).

Alternatives to the Denver test have been examined in a few LAMI countries. India has a relative wealth of research on instruments for developmental screening (Vazir et al., 1994a, 1994b) and a number of instruments have emerged. For example, the Woodside Screening Technique, which is used in India was developed in the United Kingdom (Gupta & Patel, 1991). The authors also compared the Woodside Screening Technique to the DDST and reported superior sensitivity (83%) and specificity (88%) and comparable over-referral and under-referral rates. The Baroda Developmental Screening Test was developed by choosing 31 mental and 22 motor items from the Baroda norms (Phatak et al., 1991). The Trivandrum Developmental Screening Chart, which is also derived from the Baroda norms, has 17 items (Nair et al., 1991). Unfortunately, both instruments were validated against the DDST, which itself has only moderate validity in comparison with gold standard measures that involve in- depth developmental assessment techniques (Glascoe et al., 1992). Vazir et al. (1994) developed a screening test battery for assessment of psychosocial development. This instrument, known as the Indian Council of Medical Research (ICMR) Developmental Screening Scale, was standardized on a large sample of over 13 000 urban and rural children in three regions of India. All of these instruments rely on child testing as well as caregiver reports of achievement of milestones, and are important contributions to developmental monitoring in the health system in India.

In Nigeria, a Developmental Screening Inventory (DSI) has been developed for children aged 0–30 months and a validity study has been conducted in comparison with the Bayley Scales of Infant Development. A standardization of this instrument has not yet been reported. Furthermore, it is difficult to ascertain its validity, as sensitivity and specificity values have not been reported (Aina & Morakinyo, 2001, 2005).

An instrument referred to as the Comprehensive Developmental Inventory for Infants and Toddlers has been developed in China (Province of Taiwan). Data on reliability are limited, and no data are available on the validity of the instrument compared with standard diagnostic assessments. Also, the benefits of its use within health systems have not been demonstrated (Liao & Pan, 2005; Liao et al., 2005). All of the above instruments rely on child testing methods.

As seen from the results of the DDEC Survey and the existing literature, none of these instruments is being widely used. If developmental monitoring is to become available to children worldwide, it is important to consider what kind of instruments should best be employed. In choosing a method for monitoring of child development and early detection of developmental difficulties by health providers in LAMI countries, it is important to address the following issues.

a) The generally low level of caregiver education and literacy limit the use of written questionnaires that need to be completed by the caregiver.

b) Evidence suggests that checklists about milestones and caregiver concerns may not be sufficient to identify developmental delays in LAMI countries (de Lourdes Drachler et al., 2005; Theeranate & Chuengchitraks, 2005). In populations where many children have delayed development, caregivers may not have a reference for how children should develop.

c) Caregivers may not readily express concerns or admit that their child has not reached a certain milestone if they receive health care only sporadically, do not receive health care from the same trusted provider at each visit, do not believe that interventions exist, or are concerned about stigma related to developmental difficulties (Logan, 1995).

d) Reliance on child-testing methods that involve direct elicitation of developmental skills is neither practical nor desirable in developing countries. This is partly because it is difficult and time-consuming to elicit optimal functioning of young children during health care visits. In addition, testing of a child most often leaves the caregiver watching rather than participating in the evaluation, and therefore does not

> **The method used for developmental monitoring in developing countries needs to be: (a) family-centred; (b) scientifically reliable and valid; (c) appropriate for use in various cultures; (d) brief, user-friendly, easy to learn and administer, and with minimal space requirements for documentation.**

capitalize on the partnership of clinicians with caregivers. Caregivers know their children best and, even more than in developed countries, may be the key resource to support children's development.

e) Objects are often needed to elicit skills and the cleanliness of such objects may be a major concern in developing countries.

In summary, the method used for developmental monitoring in developing countries needs to be: (a) family-centred; (b) scientifically reliable and valid; (c) appropriate for use in various cultures; (d) brief, user-friendly, easy to learn and administer, and with minimal space requirements for documentation. An example of such an instrument, which has been developed in Turkey, is described below (see page XX) (Ertem et al., 2008).

3. How should standard reference points be determined in developing countries?

Readers are referred to other reviews for details of the processes required to translate and adapt instruments for use in different populations (Peña, 2007; van Widenfelt et al., 2005). Here, particular emphasis is given to the standardization process for defining the developmental milestones. Two contrasting approaches have been used to select the population that constitutes the standard reference. In the United States, most studies using instruments that measure cognition, such as the Wechsler Intelligence Scale for Children (Wechsler, 1991) and the Bayley Scales of Infant Development (Bayley, 2006), have been conducted on population-based samples, with no attempt to exclude children with health conditions that pose risks to development. Since children in LAMI countries have much higher rates of such health conditions, however, a different approach is needed. WHO recommends that, in populations with a high prevalence of conditions that are hazardous to child health and development (such as malnutrition, low birth weight, chronic infections, parasitic infestations, iron-deficiency anaemia and perinatal complications), references for monitoring growth and development should be based on a "prescriptive sample" of healthy children without these risks, rather than on a geographical population (Borghi et al., 2006; de Onis, Garza & Victora, 2003; de Onis et al., 2006; Wijnhoven et al., 2004). This approach was applied by WHO to construct the recently launched International Growth Standards and in the WHO Motor Development Study (Wijnhoven et al., 2004). An additional contribution of these studies has been to show that, when child health is homogeneous and optimal, child growth and motor development are similar in countries with diverse conditions. The "prescriptive sample" approach is now being applied in developing countries, as exemplified by the standardization study for developmental milestones in Argentina (Lejarraga et al., 2002) and in the development of the guide for monitoring child development in Turkey (Ertem et al., 2008).

4. Do norms for developmental milestones need to be developed for every population?

This question relates to whether healthy young children attain key functional developmental milestones at similar ages. This is a question of critical importance, given the methodological and financial difficulties of standardizing developmental tests where there is little infrastructure to support the necessary studies. If young children in optimal health attain key functional developmental milestones at comparable ages around the world, then similar developmental milestones could be used worldwide, without the need for separate norms for every population.

It has long been assumed that the development of young children is different in different populations and cannot be monitored using universal standards. Earlier studies pointed to minor differences in the development of children from different backgrounds. In Jerusalem, a study of Israeli children under 12 months of age with a variety of ethnic backgrounds revealed differences in the developmental quotients: children of North African origin scored highest and those of European origin scored lowest on an adaptation of the Gessell developmental schedule (Ivanans, 1975). Keefer et al. (1982) found differences between small samples of Kenyan and American newborns on the Brazelton Neonatal Behavioral Assessment Scale, and concluded that culture-specific models of development were needed.

As a result, many countries have developed their own milestones for developmental screening tests. For example, the "restandardization" of the Denver Developmental Screening Test started in the Phillippines in 1977 (Williams, 1984). Since then the Denver test has been restandardized or adapted in Japan (Ueda, 1978), China (Song, Zhu & Gu, 1982), Turkey (Yalaz & Epir, 1983), Israel (Shapira & Harel, 1983), Indonesia (Hariyono, et al, 1987), Malaysia (Chen, 1989), India (Phatak & Khurana, 1991), Armenia (Akaragian & Dewa, 1992), Singapore (Lim, Chan & Yoong, 1994), Thailand (Sriyaporn, Pissasoontorn & Sakdisawadi, 1994), North Africa and the Eastern Mediterranean (al Naquib et al, 1999), Brazil (Drachler, Marshall, & de Carvalho Leite, 2007) and Malawi (Gladstone et al., 2008). Thousands of children in these countries were screened using the Denver test. Although vast resources were devoted to these standardization studies, the implementation of developmental monitoring during health care visits remains a problem in many of these countries. This historical overview of the standardization of the Denver test in many resource-poor countries demonstrates the need to determine whether more appropriate methods can be found to monitor child development, and whether there can be a universal set of standardized milestones.

Efforts led by WHO to identify appropriate methods to monitor child development date back to 1983. In a collaborative study in China, India and Thailand, 28 139 children were tested to define age ranges for the attainment of developmental milestones. This initiative was not designed to develop an instrument for developmental monitoring, and did not answer the critical question of whether enough similarities could be found across populations for the construction of a common monitoring instrument. The published results of this study (Lansdown, 1996) have been further investigated for this review, to improve our understanding of differences between populations of young children. The investigation found only minor differences between countries in the ages at which children attain many developmental milestones. The ages of attainment of ten developmental milestones for children under 2 years were compared for the three countries in the WHO study and for the Turkish standardization sample for the GMCD (Ertem et al, 2008). The median values reported were similar in all four countries. Although language development may be expected to be most diverse between countries, the median value for the milestone "saying one word," for example, was 9.3 months in urban China, 9.7 months in urban India and 10.2 months in Turkey. If normative development is defined on the basis of the age at which 90% or 95% of healthy children attain a particular milestone, there are likely to be few differences between countries.

The WHO Motor Development Study demonstrated that early motor development is similar across countries and that one standard can be constructed (Wijnhoven et al., 2004). Conceptually, based on innate biological and psychosocial processes, it appears that there are enough similarities in functional development between children from different ethnic, geographical or cultural backgrounds to allow one standard to be constructed for children aged 0–3 years. A multicultural study designed to confirm this, similar to that conducted for international growth curves (de Onis et al., 2003), could bring about a major advance and eliminate the need for costly and time-consuming standardization and validation of instruments for each country. It should be noted, however, that methods for developmental monitoring used in such a study should: (a) incorporate the latest information on developmental monitoring, rather than screening; (b) be culturally appropriate for use in LAMI countries; (c) be linked directly to services for developmental support and management of problems detected.

5. Is early detection of behavioural and social–emotional difficulties possible through the health system?

Developmental monitoring should include not only motor, cognitive and language development but also social–emotional development and behaviour. Indeed, current knowledge about child development brings the social–emotional domain to the forefront. Research has demonstrated that social–emotional development during the early years is a key element for good mental health and functioning in later years. Thus, the detection of social–emotional and behavioural difficulties in young children is extremely important. In the United States, the prevalence of psychosocial and behavioural problems in children has been reported to be between 12% and 27% (Briggs-Gowan et al., 2000; Cassidy & Jellinek, 1998; Simonian, 2006; Williams et al., 2004). Despite this high prevalence, the early detection of social–emotional and behavioural difficulties is inadequate. Because of lack of training and limited time during health visits, health professionals are not routinely monitoring children for behavioural and social–emotional difficulties, even in high-income countries (Cassidy & Jellinek, 1998, Reijneveld et al., 2004; Simonian, 2006). Nevertheless, it is important to note that there have been advances in instruments for monitoring social–emotional

> Conceptually, based on innate biological and psychosocial processes, it appears that there are enough similarities in functional development between children from different ethnic, geographical or cultural backgrounds to allow one standard to be constructed for children aged 0–3 years.

development within health care settings (Simonian, 2006; Weitzman & Leventhal, 2006). A review of such instruments is available and may be a useful resource for clinicians in LAMI countries (Weitzman & Leventhal, 2006).

In developing countries, although research on the behaviour and psychosocial health of children dates back to the 1970s (Minde, 1977), there has been very limited research on monitoring of social–emotional and behavioural difficulties in young children in health systems. Studies on the behavioural development of very young children have mostly aimed to determine prevalence rather than to institute a monitoring system. One study of instruments for older children has been conducted in Nigeria. This study evaluated the screening properties of the Children's Behaviour Questionnaire (CBQ) and the Reporting Questionnaire for Children (RQC) in an urban primary care setting. It showed that the two instruments were equally able to differentiate children with a specific psychiatric disorder from those without. While the CBQ was able to differentiate between conduct and emotional disorders, the RQC had the advantage of being relatively short (Omigbodun et al., 1996).

As stated by Weitzman & Leventhal (2006), "health care settings have the potential to be an optimal environment to address behavioral health concerns due to the frequent contact and trusted relationship many families have with their health providers. There is new evidence that behavioral health monitoring can be thoughtfully implemented and that system change around the detection of behavioral health problems is possible." Health systems in LAMI countries may also choose to broaden their potential and incorporate the monitoring of the social–emotional development of infants and young children into their health care practices.

6. How could health systems implement developmental monitoring?

Health systems that aim to detect developmental difficulties early will need to identify the best approaches to implementing regular developmental monitoring during routine health care services at community clinics. Developmental monitoring will need to be implemented on a broad basis for all children, and must be sustainable. Information is needed on three aspects of implementation and sustainability: (a) strategies used by community clinicians to incorporate routine developmental monitoring into health services; (b) whether the introduction of a specific instrument or training programme into community health centres increases rates of developmental monitoring and detection of developmental difficulties; and (c) whether, after training, community clinicians can reliably carry out monitoring.

Developmental monitoring may not currently be a priority for many clinicians, and there are significant potential barriers to introducing it into clinical practice. In addition, there has been very little research on how developmental monitoring can be incorporated into clinical health care practice in LAMI countries. What little research has been conducted indicates that clinicians require training in counselling caregivers on child development (Baird & Hall, 1985) and in detecting and managing developmental difficulties (Bhatia & Joseph, 2000; Figueiras et al., 2003; Kalra, Seth & Sapra, 2005; Lian et al., 2003). The North Carolina Assuring Better Child Health and Development (ABCD) project, which successfully implemented developmental monitoring in a community in the United States, may be a useful model for similar efforts in developing countries (Earls & Hay, 2006). The roadmap developed for this project shows how health providers in a clinic can work as a team to: (1) assess current protocols and practices in developmental monitoring, (2) identify a "clinician champion" in the clinic to maintain the initiative as a priority, (3) study in detail how developmental monitoring can be implemented in the clinic, (4) map the workflow, (5) identify outside support systems (such as community-based rehabilitation programmes), (6) plan staff orientations, making sure that all staff take part in the monitoring process, and (7) develop a method of collecting and sharing process and outcome data at regular intervals.

An example from a developing country

The Guide for Monitoring Child Development (GMCD) was designed in Turkey to address the need for methods to monitor the development of children in developing countries. Research in Turkey has assessed the inter-rater reliability and validity of the instrument in comparison with the Bayley Scales of Infant Development, 2nd edition (Ertem et al., 2008). A large multicountry study, supported by the United States National Institute of Health (NIH), on the international standardization, validation and efficacy of the GMCD is under way in Argentina, India, South Africa and Turkey. The conceptualization and administration of the GMCD are summarized below.

1. Conceptualization of the GMCD

The GMCD is a practical method that aims to introduce concepts of developmental monitoring and early childhood development into health care delivery systems in developing countries. The GMCD has been constructed along similar lines to the WHO/UNICEF Care for Child Development Intervention, which was summarized in Chapter 5. Health care providers can use these two methods in conjunction to monitor a child's development, using a family-centred approach, and can counsel the caregiver on how to promote the child's development. The GMCD training also includes a component on management of developmental difficulties, which aims to enable health care providers to: (a) determine the causes of developmental difficulties, (b) prevent potentiating risks factors, (c) identify protective factors, and (d) provide feedback to the caregivers on how to manage the difficulties, including giving referrals for other assessments or services.

The GMCD uses three frameworks. First, the theoretical framework of the GMCD is based on the ecological and transactional conceptualizations of child development (Forsyth, 2000; 2003), family-centred child health care (Forsyth et al., 1996), and relationship- and strengths-based developmental assessment (Wirz et al., 2005). In this approach, child development is understood, supported and managed in partnership with the family and community. Health care providers and policy-makers are consulted to identify the community's strengths, challenges, specific needs and services and to build partnerships. Second, the GMCD model views child development during the early years as a component of the life cycle approach (described in Chapter 4), which begins before conception and continues throughout the life course. The training on the GMCD emphasizes possible interventions through the health care system, for example preconceptional interventions such as family planning. Third, the GMCD includes functional development, so that the child's health and development can be addressed within the framework of the WHO International Classification of Functioning for Children and Youth (Lollar & Simeonsson, 2005). Health care providers trained in using the GMCD can obtain information that can be applied to the WHO ICF model, which describes children's health and well-being in terms of four components: (1) body structures, (2) body functions, (3) activities, and (4) participation. The GMCD, therefore, is not merely a screening test, but a system for monitoring child development within the health service, which can be seamlessly linked to systems for promotion of child development and for prevention and management of developmental difficulties.

2. Administration of the GMCD

The GMCD provides a method for developmental monitoring and early detection of developmental difficulties that is easy for health care providers to learn and apply during a health encounter.

The GMCD is an open-ended, precoded, 10-minute interview with the primary caregiver of a child aged under 42 months. The interview technique:

- builds on patient-centred communication techniques in medicine (Boyle, Dwinnell & Platt, 2005; Teutsch, 2003);

- is based on the fundamental principles of human communication and recall of information (Fisher & McCauley, 1995);

- catalyses communication between clinicians and caregivers, while obtaining an overview of the child's development;

- avoids "socially desirable" answers and assumptions about what the child should be doing and

- is designed to be as culturally neutral as possible.

Caregivers are first given an explanation of the reason for the interview and their interest and cooperation are elicited.

The questions to be asked when administering the GMCD, together with the milestones for two of the age ranges, are shown in Table 2. The first question is adapted from Glascoe's Parent's Evaluation of Developmental Status (PEDS) (Glascoe, 2002) and seeks to identify parental concerns. If the caregiver expresses concerns, these are explored further before moving on to the other questions. If the caregiver does not have concerns, the clinician explains the importance of obtaining a portrayal of the child's typical functioning and asks the open-ended questions 2–7. If necessary, prompts may be used to explain the questions. The seven questions are related to the following developmental domains: (1) caregiver concerns in any area of development, (2) expressive language, (3) receptive language, (4) fine and gross motor functions, (5) social–emotional and relational functions, (6) play, and (7) self-help skills (for children older than 12 months). The GMCD does not

Table 2. Questions to be asked when administering the GMCD and examples of functional milestones

Developmental domain and interview questions	Functional milestones at age: 6–7 months	Functional milestones at age: 8–10 months
1. Concerns. "By "development", I mean learning, understanding, communicating, relationships, behaviour and emotions, how your child uses her fingers and hands, legs and body, hearing and vision. Do you have any concerns about your child's development in any of these areas?"		
2. Expressive language and communication. "Tell me about how your child communicates. How does she let you know when she wants something?"	Makes "ga, gu, da, bı," sounds (joins vowels and consonants).	Repeats syllables like "da-da" Uses gestures like shaking head in protest
3. Receptive language. "Tell me examples of what she can understand when you talk to her?"	When caregiver speaks, child listens, looks at her mouth Recognizes and prefers caregiver's voice Responds with sounds when talked to	Understands repeated simple words like "mummy", "no".
4. Fine and gross motor functions. What does [child's name] do with her hands and fingers, and with her legs and body?"	Reaches with hands. Holds on to toys or objects Sits with support Bears weight on legs	Transfers objects from hand to hand Picks up small objects, like raisins Rolls from front to back Sits without support
5. Relationship (social-emotional). "Tell me about your child's relationships with people she knows. What about strangers? How does she relate to them?"	Recognizes caregivers, reaches to them, smiles, inspects their faces	Reacts when mother leaves May turn away from strangers in anxiety, caution, shyness or fear
6. Play (social-emotional, cognitive). "I'd like to learn about how she plays. Can you give me some examples?"	Regards hands Shakes objects Responds to "peek-a-boo"	Inspects toys with curiosity Throws, bangs toys, objects Looks for objects Plays "peek-a-boo"
7. Self-help skills. "What kinds of things can [child's name] do for herself now, like eating or dressing?"		

have separate questions for the cognitive domain, as it is difficult for caregivers of young children to describe cognitive skills separate from the above domains. Cognitive functions are involved in these domains, and the first question specifically asks if the caregiver has concerns about the child's learning.

The outcome of the monitoring is a form, comprising two tables, with the questions in the rows and the age ranges in the columns. The age ranges were selected to correspond to the health monitoring and immunization schedules recommended by WHO. The cells contain developmental milestones, constructed using five previously standardized and validated developmental screening or assessment instruments: Denver II (Frankenburg et al., 1992), Vineland (Sparrow, Balla & Cicchetti, 1984), Brigance Screening Test (Glascoe, 1996), Ages and Stages Questionnaire (Bricker et al., 1995), and Bayley Scales of Infant Development, 2nd edition (Bayley II) (Bayley, 1993), as well as extensive interviews with caregivers of young children. The standard ages for attainment of the milestones were based on a prescriptive sample of 505 healthy Turkish children aged 0–2 years. In two clinical samples, the inter-rater reliability between medical students and a child development specialist, and the validity of the GMCD administered during a health visit in comparison with a comprehensive developmental assessment with the Bayley II, were examined. Inter-rater agreement, as measured by kappa, as well as sensitivity, specificity, and positive and negative predictive values, was found to be above 0.84.

In conclusion, the GMCD is an innovative method for monitoring child development that is designed specifically for use by health care providers in developing countries. Studies in Turkey have provided preliminary evidence for its reliability and validity. The training can be completed in three days; the training package consists of written materials, slides and demonstration videos. Recently the GMCD has received both national and international recognition. All three components of the package have been adopted by the Turkish Ministry of Health and UNICEF Turkey for use in a nationwide training programme on child development for primary health care providers. There is growing interest among clinicians and researchers from Algeria, Australia, Eritrea, Georgia, India, Pakistan, South Africa and Zambia in using the GMCD training in the early detection and management of children with developmental difficulties.

Conclusions and implications for action

1. The DDEC Survey found that standardized methods for the early detection of developmental difficulties are not widely used.

2. Developmental monitoring, using a family-centred, comprehensive approach during health care encounters, is used in many high-income countries as an effective method for the early detection of developmental difficulties.

3. The family's active partnership during the monitoring process and a continuous relationship between the clinician and the family are key to the early detection of developmental difficulties.

4. Developmental monitoring must be comprehensive and clinically relevant, so that multiple aspects of the child's health and development and the family's needs and functioning are taken into consideration, rather than just the results of a screening test.

5. Conceptually contemporary, clinically appropriate, scientifically reliable and valid instruments should be used for developmental monitoring, rather than non-standard approaches. The "prescriptive sample" approach of the WHO should be used to develop standard reference values. Whether each new instrument needs to be restandardized for every population is a question that needs to be addressed.

6. Screening for identifiable and treatable conditions, such as iron deficiency, hearing loss, and metabolic, genetic, infectious or other disorders should be integrated into developmental monitoring.

7. The early detection of developmental difficulties should allow a seamless transition to services that will support the child's development when needed.

Chapter 7

Developmental assessment of young children

DDEC Survey results

In the DDEC Survey, questions 15 and 16 were specifically related to developmental assessment (see Annex 1). In most countries, the paediatrician or community health provider conducted a developmental assessment and diagnosed developmental difficulties. Similarly, in most countries, the paediatrician decided which kinds of early intervention or rehabilitation services the children should receive.

Purpose of chapter and additional key references

As described in Chapter 6, the early detection of developmental difficulties is possible through developmental monitoring during health care encounters. Children with such difficulties should then be comprehensively assessed to establish a diagnosis and ascertain their level of functioning, in order to determine their needs for additional support and services and to enable them to obtain such services. This chapter provides information on the basic principles of the developmental evaluation of young children with suspected developmental difficulties. The intention is to provide information on the types of developmental assessment that are desirable and how to begin the process of building infrastructure for such assessments.

Often in developed countries, teams of clinicians with various backgrounds evaluate the child and the family. These clinicians may have a background in developmental–behavioural paediatrics, paediatric neurology, child psychiatry, early intervention, child pyschology, child development, audiology, speech therapy, special education, occupational therapy, physical therapy and rehabilitation, ophthalmology, orthopaedics or clinical genetics. In countries with fewer resources, children may be evaluated by one or a few clinicians with backgrounds in one of these disciplines. The discrepancy between developing and developed countries may dishearten clinicians working in such resource-poor settings. It may appear that, because of the limited number and variety of clinicians available, "state of the art" developmental assessments cannot be conducted. The principles of developmental assessment, however, can be successfully applied by any experienced clinician in any setting. On the other hand, when these principles are not applied, even if many clinicians working in multidisciplinary teams conduct the assessment, the child and the family may not be fully understood and therefore not helped.

A detailed description of a comprehensive developmental assessment is beyond the scope of this chapter. Readers are referred to an excellent book by Meisels & Fenichel (1996), two renowned leaders in the field of early childhood development. The book describes in detail multiple aspects of the guidelines for developmental assessment. Key components of family-centred assessment can also be found in books on early intervention by Guralnick (2005a) and Shonkoff & Meisels (2000).

Conceptualization

As a summary of contemporary visions for developmental assessment, ten key components have been distilled from multiple sources.

1. **The assessment should be based on the principles of family-centred care.** "Family-centred" means that the family or caregivers of the child and the professionals who are conducting the evaluation are partners in the evaluation (Committee on Hospital Care, American Academy of Pediatrics, 2003). The family provides information about the child's functioning, strengths, vulnerabilities and needs for support, as well as their own concerns, needs and what they have accomplished and how. The consulting pro-

fessional conducts the evaluation together with the family, providing the expertise to help the child and family recognize their strengths and areas of need, and suggesting interventions that could help the child reach an optimum level of functioning. Results of the assessment are not "given" to the caregivers; on the contrary, the assessment is a process during which the caregivers and the clinician discover the results together. The reason for the assessment, the details of how the assessment will be carried out and the role of the caregivers as partners in the assessment should be shared with the family. The key elements of family-centred assessment can be defined as respect for the capacity of the child and family and humility about the process of helping them. In this process, the most effcetive clinician, regardless of profession or background, is the one who knows that he or she is learning together with the family, that answers lie within the strengths of the child, the family and the community, and that his or her role is to help the family recognize and use these strengths in a supportive and caring assessment process.

2. **The assessment should be comprehensive and include all aspects of the child's development.** The assessment should incorporate: physical health, growth, vision and hearing, and special laboratory tests that may be warranted to detect biological causes of developmental difficulties (particularly anaemia, malnutrition and chronic infections in LAMI countries). The family's composition, physical and mental health and functioning, social support systems within the larger family or community, and the nurturing and stimulation provided in the home environment are crucial elements of the assessment. Furthermore, the clinician should explore what the caregivers have already done to support the child's development, what they understand about the specific needs of the child, their concerns, fears, hopes and desires, and their knowledge of community resources.

3. **Identification of caregiver concerns should form a crucial component of the interview.** A review of caregivers' concerns provides an important starting-point for developmental assessment. If caregivers raise concerns, the clinician will need to observe these areas of development in more detail during the assessment, and caregivers' questions should be addressed. Asking about concerns also enables the clinician to determine how well the caregivers have observed the child and what is important to them in their child's development. When caregivers share their concerns with the clinician, this can serve as a starting-point for providing feedback.

4. **The clinician should obtain a detailed developmental history, so that risks and protective factors in the life of the child and the family and the child's past progress or deterioration can be determined.** Ideally, the history should begin from the childhood of the caregivers and their upbringing, and should include all relevant information about the child and family, their past and present functioning, and future aspirations.

5. **Observations of the child's interactions with his or her caregivers are fundamental to the developmental assessment.** More important than standardized testing, observations of the child in a free-play environment will provide invaluable information on functional development.

6. **Information on the nurturing and stimulation provided in the home environment and daily life of the child is indispensable.** If this part of the evaluation can be conducted in the home, it will provide the most reliable and valid information about the child's development. In many countries, home visits by health care providers are well accepted. In many early intervention programmes around the world, health clinicians are trained to conduct a home visit, which includes an interview with caregivers and observations of the child and family in a natural setting. If a home visit is not possible, the assessment should at least include questions related to the daily life of the child and how the child is cared for, nurtured and stimulated in the home. The interview should also give caregivers a chance to discuss their perceptions of the caregiving. For example, the clinician can ask whether caregivers think that the child is getting enough nurturing and stimulation or whether they have concerns.

7. **Identification of the social supports of the caregivers and family is also an important element.** The support systems that the family has – or does not have – may be key factors in determining whether the family will be able to enhance the child's development.

8. **The mental and physical health of the caregivers is key to the development of the child.** It should be determined in every developmental assessment.

9. **Formal developmental assessment instruments provide a structure for the interactions between the clinician and the child and family.** The child and family will obtain most benefit from these instruments if they are used to identify the child's and family's strengths and the areas of development that need support. The clinician should not rely on developmental screening tests (such as those listed in Chapter 6). Such tests are designed to detect developmental difficulties early but not to provide in-depth information about functioning or areas that need support. More detailed assessment instruments and techniques which are explained in the next section needed.

   Regardless of the technique, the key principle in applying instruments is to use them within a family-centred framework. If instruments are used mechanically, in a testing environment, by an examiner who does not know the child and whom the child and family do not know, the testing will often be meaningless. Instruments should be used in the presence of the caregiver and with his or her assistance. The fine and gross motor, cognitive, language and social–emotional skills of a young child may be important at the time of evaluation. Equally important, however, are functions that will enable the child to develop further. Together with the caregiver, the clinician can use standard test objects and play materials to obtain an understanding of, for example, attention span, engagement with people and objects, interest in the environment, capacity to initiate interactions and play, engagement in purposeful interactions and behaviour, problem-solving skills, temperament, curiosity, and ability to deal with frustration and regulate emotions.

   Developmental test scores can be useful for research purposes, to provide means and standard deviations for samples and populations. However, they are often not meaningful when applied to individual children in a clinical context. The clinician should be able to interpret test scores for the family, avoiding any negative consequences of using such scores, such as the stigmatization of children with "suboptimal" scores.

10. **The developmental assessment of the child should be seamlessly linked with interventions to address developmental difficulties.** In fact, the assessment should be viewed as the first component of an intervention. Information on what the family has already tried, the services and treatments that they have sought, their expectations of other interventions, and their level of information on how to access services should be determined. The clinician should identify, in conjunction with the family, the kinds of services the child and family need and what is available in the community. If necessary, additional resources should be sought together with the family.

The above guidelines highlight the core principles of developmental assessment. The clinician conducting the assessment – regardless of his or her background – should be trained in the core principles of child development and family-centred care and experienced in clinical therapeutic practices. The assessment is best conducted using a "transdisciplinary" model (Magill-Evans, Hodge & Darrah, 2002). In this model, one clinician takes on primary responsibility for the child and family. This clinician, working across disciplines, can then seek information about specific aspects of the child's or family's difficulties by consulting written materials or experts in related disciplines. The transdisciplinary approach is regarded by many child development specialists as more appropriate than the multidisciplinary model, where the child and family may feel confused because they have to deal with multiple experts with whom they do not necessarily have a relationship of trust. The transdisciplinary approach is also likely to be more appropriate for LAMI countries, where there are few trained professionals.

Research in LAMI countries

Assessment processes

There have been very few studies of the process of developmental assessment in developing countries. An important study in South Africa in the 1990s shed light on the importance of family-centred assessment (Venter, 1997a). Before and after their first visit to a neurodevelopmental outpatient clinic, caregivers were interviewed about their understanding of their child's disability and their expectations of the service offered at the clinics. Before the consultation, the majority of caregivers had a fair understanding of the child's functional problems and the short-term complications. Surprisingly, after the consultation, levels of understanding were reported to have decreased significantly. Caregivers, however, had a significantly improved understanding of the etiology of the problem, while their understanding of long-term complications did not differ significantly before and after the consultation.

In a more recent study in Israel (Lavi & Rosenberg, 2005), parents whose children first received a diagnosis of mental retardation, autism or pervasive developmental disorder (PDD), cerebral palsy, or genetic syndromes were asked for feedback on their experience in being informed of their child's disability. A self-report survey questionnaire was mailed to the caregivers, to be completed anonymously. Questions were based on a survey of the literature and focused on the setting of the meeting, its contents, staff behaviour, and parents' satisfaction with the meeting; information on background characteristics of the family and child was also obtained. Approximately two-thirds (63%) of respondents reported a high level of satisfaction with the meeting at which they first heard the diagnosis. Content analysis of open questions and statistical analysis of correlations between satisfaction and a series of potential predictors pointed to three main areas that affected parental satisfaction.

1. The amount and type of information conveyed. Parental satisfaction was higher when detailed information was provided about a number of issues (diagnosis, treatment options, educational settings, rights for benefits and assistance etc.), when parents were referred to additional sources of information, and when the clinician was seen to be knowledgeable and confident.

2. Attitudes of staff regarding the child's condition. Parental satisfaction was higher when the child's strengths (and not only problems) were addressed, when the general tone was not pessimistic and hope and optimism were also conveyed, and when expected and possible future developments were specified.

3. Staff approach to the parents. Parental satisfaction was higher when staff were attentive and empathic, when they clearly expressed willingness to accompany and assist the family over time, when they were respectful towards the parents and related to them as equal partners, and when parents felt that they had been informed of the diagnosis without delay and that no information had been withheld.

A study in Zimbabwe indicated that caregiver concerns, such as social stigmatization, feelings of isolation and emotional pain, take precedence over the child's difficulties in the initial assessment (House, McAlister & Naidoo, 1990).

Two studies, in the Libyan Arab Jamahiriya and Turkey, demonstrated the importance of a comprehensive evaluation. In the Libyan Arab Jamahiriya, many children with cerebral palsy were found to have undiagnosed and unaddressed cognitive developmental difficulties (Khan, 1992). The Turkish study revealed that neuroimaging techniques and genetic and metabolic testing could identify the causal factors in 43% of children with significant developmental difficulties (Ozmen et al., 2005). This was a tertiary-care sample of children with severe difficulties. It should be noted that tertiary-care-based laboratory techniques, when conducted indiscriminately, will often not identify causal factors for developmental difficulties in young children in LAMI countries. It is more important to determine the causes of treatable underlying disorders, such as understimulation in the home environment, malnutrition, anaemia, chronic infections or infestations, and hearing loss due to otitis media.

There is very little information from developing countries on the role of clinicians from different disciplines. The role of psychologists has been emphasized in one report from a child development centre in Israel (Tirosh, Amit & Harel, 1999).

Similarly, research is greatly needed in developing countries on how to improve the understanding of caregivers of the implications of a developmental assessment. In one innovative approach in England, for example, parents were given a videotape summary of their child's assessment. This method was favoured by 89% of Urdu- and Punjabi-speaking (immigrant) parents and 43% of English-speaking parents. The method, however, did not lead to improved recall of the summary's content six weeks later (Ilett, 1995).

Assessment instruments

Instruments for developmental assessment take much more time and resources to develop, adapt and standardize than instruments for developmental screening or monitoring. As a result, very few assessment instruments have been developed and standardized in developing countries. Table 3 lists a number of instruments that can be used to assess components of development together with published research using these instruments in

Table 3. Examples of instruments for developmental assessment and related research in developing countries

Component of assessment	Instruments that can be used to assess the component	Research from developing countries using these instruments
Comprehensive developmental interview	Diagnostic Instrument for Children and Adolescents (DICA)	Ethiopia (Ashenafi et al., 2000, 2001)
Nurturing and stimulation in home environment	Home Observation for Measurement of the Environment (HOME) (Bradley & Caldwell, 1977) Supplement to the HOME for Impoverished Families (SHIF) (Ertem et al., 1997)	Bangladesh (Black et al., 2007) Brazil (Andrade et al., 2005) United Republic of Tanzania (Mbise & Kysela, 1990)
Family competence and social support	Family Support Scale Parent Needs Survey (Seligman & Benjamin Darling, 1989) Parenting Stress Index (Abidin, 1983)	China (Ngai, Wai Chi Chan & Holroyd, 2007)
Caregiver mental health	Edinburgh Postnatal Depression Scale (EPDS)	Bangladesh (Black et al., 2007) Islamic Republic of Iran (Montazeri, Torkan & Omidvari, 2007) China (Lee et al., 1998) UK-based South Asian women (Downe, Butler & Hinder, 2007) South Africa (Lawrie et al., 1998)
Functional development	Non-structured play PEDI Vineland Scales of Adaptive Behavior	Egypt (Wachs et al., 1993) Turkey (Erkin et al., 2007) Singapore (Agarwal et al., 2005) Indonesia (Tombokan-Runtukahu & Nitko, 1992)
Cognitive development	Bayley Scales of Infant Development, Bayley II or Bayley III	Israel (Horowitz et al., 1977) Bangladesh (Black et al., 2007, Hamadani et al., 2002; Khan et al., 2006) India (Chaudhari et al., 1990, 1995) Brazil (Andrade et al., 2005, Eickmann et al., 2007; Grantham McGregor et al., 1998) Chile (Castillo-Durán et al., 2001; Vega et al., 1999) Bolivia (Bender et al., 1994) United Republic of Tanzania (McGrath et al., 2006) Nigeria (Aina & Morakinyo, 2005) Kenya (Bhargava, 2000; Neumann et al., 1991; Whaley et al., 1998) Uganda (Drotar et al., 1999) Zimbabwe (Wolf et al., 1997; 1999) South Africa (Cooper & Sandler, 1997) Ethiopia (Aboud & Alemu, 1995; Kirksey et al., 1994; Young et al., 1982)
Language development	Reynell Language Development Scales (Reynell, 1979) Symbolic Play Test (SPT) (Lowe and Costello, 1976; Udwin & Yule, 1982)	China, Hong Kong SAR (Au et al., 2004) China (Chu et al., 2006)
Instruments for children with visual difficulties	Reynell-Zinkin Scales (Reynell, 1979)	Bangladesh (Khan et al., 2006)

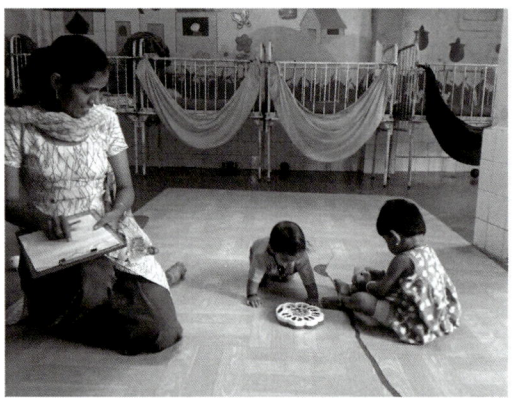

Comprehensive assessment requires providers trained in early childhood development: children assessed by Child Development Aide, India. Photo: Dr. Vibha Krishnamurthy

populations from developing countries. Although there have been a number of studies, the most informative component of the assessment – the developmental interview – has received little attention. Ashenafi et al. (2000, 2001) used the Diagnostic Instrument for Chidren and Adolescents (DICA) to assess developmental and psychosocial problems in children. Most research, however, has focused on assessment of cognitive and motor development, usually using the Bayley Scales of Infant Development.

Whether instruments for developmental assessment need to be restandardized for each population remains an open question. Given that the person conducting the evaluation has to have intense training, and that most instruments take at least an hour to administer and require special conditions (such as toys and a soundproof room), the restandardizing process is a time- and resource-consuming process. Furthermore, as happened with the Bayley II and III, newer standardizations may be released from developed countries before assessment instruments can be standardized in developing countries.

Another important question is whether developing countries should allocate resources to developing their own assessment instruments. Using the norms developed in other countries should not constitute a major problem for research that aims to: (a) measure differences in developmental scores between groups of children, such as premature infants and term infants or intervention and control groups; (b) measure changes over time in a group of children. The question of whether restandardization will be necessary becomes important and relevant if the research aims to: (a) compare children's development scores between populations; (b) interpret scores in terms of what constitutes developmental delay.

A pilot study aimed to determine whether the original norms of the Miller Assessment for Preschoolers (MAP) could be used in Israel. This scale is used to evaluate preschool children with suspected problems. No significant differences were found between the Israeli sample and the US standardization sample on the MAP total score. Israeli children, however, performed below US norms on the Foundations Index, a component of the MAP that assesses abilities involving basic motor tasks and the awareness of sensations (Schneider et al., 1995).

Studies in many different countries have used assessment instruments, such as the Bayley Scales of Infant Development, with United States norms. In India, considerable research has been conducted to develop instruments for developmental assessment and screening (Chaudhari, 1996). The Bayley Scales of Infant Development have been adapted and are referred to as the Baroda norms (Phatak et al., 1991).

A multifaceted developmental test of cognitive skills was constructed in India, modelled on the Bus Puzzle Test (Egan & Brown, 1984). Pilot-tests in Rajasthan examined a simple ethnic modification of the original test, development of more socioculturally appropriate scenes, a detailed statistical procedure of item analysis and reliability studies. The picture was converted into a wooden insert puzzle, called the Indan Picture Puzzle Test (IPPT) and standardized using a random sample of 616 children. The IPPT assesses aspects of early language, picture interpretation, performance skills and conceptual development in children aged 2–5 years (Singhania & Sonksen, 2004).

The Developmental Profile II (DP II) assesses developmental status from birth to 9½ years in five domains – physical, social, self-help, academic and communication (Alpern, Boll & Shearer, 1986). The DP II has been used in India and shown to be effective in comparing developmental functioning of autistic and non-autistic children (Malhi & Singhi, 2002).

Studies in Bangladesh (Black et al., 2007), Brazil (Andrade et al., 2005) and the United Republic of Tanzania (Mbise & Kysela, 1990) used the Home Observation for Measurement of the Environment (HOME) scale to measure the effect of the nurturing and stimulation provided in the home environment on child development. Developed in the United States in the 1970s (Bradley & Caldwell, 1977), the HOME scale has been one of the most widely used instruments to measure the environmental component of the transactional model of child development. The Supplement to the HOME for Impoverished Families (SHIF) has been shown to be more effective in measuring the "lower" end of poverty, stimulation and nurturing when used in impoverished populations in developed countries. The SHIF may also be an important addition to the HOME for assessing nurturing and stimulation in developing countries (Ertem et al., 1997).

More functional aspects of development, such as adaptive functioning and play, quality of life of the child, and aspects related to the home environment or family have been less commonly assessed. Instruments for the measurement of functional skills in young children with developmental difficulties have recently been reviewed in detail (Msall, 2005). The following were included in the review: the Infant and Toddler Quality of Life Questionnaire (ITQOL), the Netherlands Office of Prevention Assessment of Preschool Quality of Life (TAPQOL), the Health Status Classification System-PreSchool (HSCS-PS), the Pediatric Evaluation of Disability Inventory (PEDI), the Vineland Adaptive Behavior Scale (VABS), the Warner Inventory of Developmental and Emerging Adaptive and Functional Skills (Warner IDEA-FS), the Scales of Independent Behavior Revised (SIB-R) Early Development Form, the Pediatric Functional Independence Measure (WeeFIM), and the Pediatric Quality of Life Inventory Version 4 (PedsQL 4.0). The PEDI has been widely used, for example in the United States (Haley et al., 2004), Sweden (Odman, Krevers & Oberg, 2007), the Netherlands (Custers et al., 2002; Vos-Vromans, Ketelaar & Gorter, 2005), Norway (Dolva, Coster & Lilja, 2004; Ostensjo et al., 2006) and China (Province of Taiwan) (Yang et al., 2003). Research using this instrument in developing areas has been limited to Turkey (Erkin et al., 2007), Slovenia (Srsen, Vidmar & Zupan, 2005) and Puerto Rico (Gannotti & Cruz, 2001). The Turkish study showed that the translated form of the PEDI had good internal consistency and reliability. Both the standardization study in Slovenia and the validation study in Puerto Rico, however, suggested that there were significant differences between cultures in their understanding and demonstration of functional skills. In particular, caregiver assistance scale scores in Slovenia were different from the American normative data, particularly in the youngest age group. Slovene children were consistently found to be different from American children at comparable ages (scoring either higher or lower) in several functional skills and caregiver assistance scales. The studies also confirmed the influence of gender and the presence of siblings on the scores of some functional skills and caregiver assistance scales. The level of parent education did not have a significant impact on the results. Further research is needed to determine whether functional measures need to be restandardized for every population.

Very few studies have used quality of life measures for young children in developing countries (Shek & Lee, 2007). A study in China, Hong Kong Special Administrative Region, using the Chinese Pediatric Quality of Life Inventory (PedsQL) found that overall well-being and psychosocial health scores were significantly lower in children with developmental difficulties (Lau, Chow & Lo, 2006).

There has been very little research in developing countries on instruments to assess children's language. In one study in China, the Symbolic Play Test (SPT), which is used to assess language skills (Lowe & Costello, 1976; Udwin & Yule, 1982), was modified for use with Chinese children (Chu et al., 2006). In another study in China, Hong Kong SAR, both the Reynell Development Language Scales (Reynell, 1979) were shown to be appropriate for use with Cantonese-speaking young children (Au et al., 2004).

Similarly, very few studies have used instruments for the developmental assessment of visually impaired (Khan et al., 2006) or hearing-impaired children (Olusanya, 2007; Olusanya & Newton, 2007).

Conclusions and implications for action

1. The DDEC Survey found that developmental difficulties in young children were assessed, diagnosed and referred for services mostly by paediatricians and primary health care providers.

2. Although LAMI countries may not have the infrastructure and resources for multidisciplinary evaluations, such as are conducted in many high-income countries to diagnose developmental difficulties, the family-centred principles of a developmental assessment can be adapted for use around the world.

3. Research on developmental assessment in LAMI countries has generally been restricted to use of various instruments. The most frequently studied aspect has been instruments for assessment of cognitive development. A range of key concepts have also been studied in LAMI countries to a limited extent. These

are: the developmental interview, assessment of nurturing and stimulation in the home environment, family competence and social support systems, family mental health, functional development of the child, and language development. There is a great shortage of research on assessment using the developmental interviewing, social and emotional, and functional assessments.

4. There is a need to develop universal systems and guidelines for developmental assessment that are anchored in current scientific information and conceptualizations of child development.

Chapter

International classification systems for developmental difficulties in young children

DDEC Survey results

Question 17 of the DDEC Survey asked what eligibility criteria were used for young children to receive early intervention services. Approximately half of the countries had such criteria. The most commonly used criteria were: a non-standard disability score or percentage of disability, a diagnosis of disability, IQ score, or a documentation of developmental delay. In only one country was the WHO manual on community-based rehabilitation (Helander, Mendis & Nelson, 1989) being used as the criteria for entry into early intervention services.

Question 12 of the DDEC Survey asked respondents to name classification systems used in their country by health care providers responsible for diagnosing or determining the presence of developmental difficulties in young children. In the vast majority of countries, classification systems were not routinely used in these contexts. The International Classification of Diseases (ICD 10 or ICD 9) was being used in four countries, and the International Classification of Functioning, Disability and Health (ICF) and the Diagnostic and Statistical Classification of Mental Disorders (DSM-IV) were each being used routinely in three countries.

Purpose and scope of the chapter and additional key resources

This chapter summarizes the systems that can be used to classify developmental difficulties in young children. Three well known systems will be summarized: the International Classification of Diseases (ICD), and the International Classification of Functioning, Disability and Health (ICF), both published by WHO (2004, 2001b); and the Diagnostic Classification of Mental Health and Developmental Disorders of Infancy and Early Childhood: revised edition (DC: 0-3R), developed by Zero to Three (2005). Readers are also referred to other key reviews on classification systems for child health and development (Msall, 2005; 2006; Simeonsson, Scarborough & Hebbeler, 2006; Stein & Silver, 1999).

Conceptualization

Classification systems can be useful in four areas of early childhood development: (a) formulation of clinical information, (b) research, (c) policy and (d) advocacy. Classification systems define the components of clinical assessment, summarize and highlight the relevant aspects of the clinical information that has been obtained, as well as information that is missing, and allow information to be shared between clinicians. The clinical use of a classification system may be overlooked, as clinicians often have a "sense" of the diagnosis and may be reluctant to attach a name and label, particularly for young children whose development is constantly evolving. Classification systems can be meaningful for clinicians, as a means of linking their individual patients with general scientific information, and of communicating with other professionals through a common language related to the etiology, epidemiology, prognosis and treatment of disorders. Classification systems may also be useful for systematizing clinical concepts, and assessing and formulating previously overlooked areas of child development (Emde & Wise, 2003; Jakob et al., 2007).

For research purposes, internationally endorsed classifications can help formulate research questions, and allow research data to be gathered, stored, analysed, retrieved and interpreted (Jakob et al., 2007).

Policy-makers and advocates may also find classification systems useful for determining which children need services, monitoring the kinds of services received by groups of children who fall within certain classifications, and advocating for additional services.

Historically, WHO has been the prime instigator of international health classification systems. The Family of International Classifications (WHO-FIC) is a set of classification products that may be used in an integrated fashion to compile and compare health information, nationally and internationally. The main systems are reference classifications, which cover the main parameters of the health system, such as death, disease, functioning, disability, health and health interventions. WHO reference classifications have received broad international acceptance and agreement for use, and are recommended for international reporting on health. WHO has developed two reference classifications that can be used to describe the health status of an individual at a particular point in time. These are the International Classification of Diseases, now in its 10th revision (ICD-10) (WHO, 2004) and the International Classification of Functioning, Disability and Health (ICF) (WHO, 2001b). The International Classification of Health Interventions (ICHI) is still under development. Both the ICD and ICF can be used alone or in conjunction (as recommended by WHO) to classify developmental status and developmental difficulties in young children. Neither of these systems, however, was specifically developed for young children. Zero to Three, the main organization for young children in the United States, has developed a system specifically to classify developmental and mental health disorders during infancy and early childhood: the Diagnostic Classification of Mental Health and Developmental Disorders of Infancy and Early Childhood, revised edition (DC: 0-3R) (Zero to Three, 2005). The strengths and the areas that need improvement in each of these systems are summarized below in a format that may be practical for clinicians, researchers, policy-makers and advocates.

The Diagnostic Classification of Mental Health and Developmental Disorders of Infancy and Early Childhood

The need for the DC: 0-3 stemmed from the inadequacy of the Diagnostic and Statistical Manual of Mental Disorders (DSM) in addressing developmental and mental health difficulties during infancy and early childhood (Zero to Three, 2005). There have been five revisions of the DSM since it was first published in 1952. The last major revision was DSM-IV (American Psychiatric Association, 1994) further "text revision" DSM-IV-TR was produced in 2000 (American Psychiatric Association, 2000). The DSM-V is currently in preparation, and is due for publication the near future. The DSM-IV is a categorical classification system. The categories are prototypes, and a patient with a close approximation to the prototype is said to have that disorder. Each category of disorder has a numerical code taken from the ICD coding system, which is used for health service administrative purposes, including insurance, as well as research.

The DC: 0-3 was published by Zero to Three in 1994, as a systematic, developmentally based approach to classification of mental health and developmental disorders in infancy and early childhood. The purpose of the DC: 0-3 was to provide a basis on which clinicians and researchers could identify, assess and classify early childhood disorders and develop appropriate treatment interventions. The DC: 0-3 aimed to create a common language among clinicians and researchers to promote better understanding of the nature of early childhood disorders. The classification system is used by professionals around the world. It is rooted in both psychodynamic and psychoanalytical traditions, including developmental, family systems, relationship, and attachment theories (Dunst, Storck & Snyder, 2006). While the DSM concentrates on pathology, the DC: 0-3 is unique in that it employs biopsychosocial and bioecological models in axis II, the relational context of the child, particularly the primary care-giving dyad (see below). A revised version of DC: 0-3, DC: 0-3R, was published in 2005 (Zero to Three, 2005). In the years since its publication, DC: 0-3 has become increasingly valued as a complement to the DSM and ICD classifications. It has been published in eight additional languages, increasing its accessibility to clinicians around the world.

The DC: 0-3 aims to complement, but not replace, the DSM and has a similar multiaxial categorization. There are five axes, all of which are given equal weight in the diagnostic process:

Axis I. Primary diagnosis. Disorders in this axis are: post-traumatic stress disorder; deprivation matreatment disorder, disorders of affect, prolonged bereavement/grief reaction, anxiety disorders, depression, adjustment disorder, regulation disorders, sleep behaviour disorder, feeding behaviour disorder, disorders of relating and communicating, multisystem developmental disorder.

Axis II. Relationship classification. This axis examines the behavioural quality of the interaction between child and caregiver, the affective tone of the dyad, and the psychological involvement between them. Relationships are classified as over-involved, under-involved, anxious/tense, angry/hostile, mixed, or abusive. The Parent-Infant Relationship Global Assessment Scale (PIR-GAS) is used to rate the nature of the care-giving dyad.

Axis III. Co-existing medical and developmental disorders. A diagnosis of developmental delay, malnutrition, infectious disease, neurological condition or hearing or visual loss would be placed here.

Axis IV. Psychosocial stressors. This axis aims to identify stressors and risk factors present in the child's environment and their overall effects on the child. Stressors may be predominantly acute or predominantly enduring, and the overall impact may be diagnosed as mild, moderate, or severe.

Axis V. Functional emotional developmental level. This axis describes six capacities that contribute to the social and emotional development of the child: attention and regulation, forming relationships and mutual engagement, intentional two-way communication, complex gestures and problem-solving, use of symbols to express thoughts and feelings, and connecting symbols logically and abstract thinking.

The International Classification of Diseases

The ICD categorizes diseases, health-related conditions and external causes of disease and injury for use in compiling mortality and morbidity statistics. The categories of the ICD are also useful for decision-support systems, reimbursement systems and documentation of medical information (WHO, 2004). The ICD had its origins in the 19th century, stemming from the need to categorize diseases for public health purposes. WHO has been responsible for the ICD since its 6th revision in 1948. With a need for comparability at the international level in both public health and clinical research, more and more clinical concepts were introduced into the ICD, resulting in its current 10th revision (WHO 2004a). An updating mechanism allows yearly updates and major revisions every 3 years. The revision process towards ICD-11 started in 2006, and publication is expected by 2015. The ICD is used in systematic mortality registration in more than 117 countries and has been translated into over 40 languages. ICD-10 is used in many countries also for morbidity coding for reimbursement, treatment and research. The classification can be viewed online in English and French at the WHO website (http://www.who.int/classifications/icd/en/) and in other languages through the relative national institutions.

International Classification of Functioning, Disability, and Health

The ICF provides a unified and standard language and framework for the description of health and health-related states of individuals. It was previously the International Classification of Impairments, Disabilities, and Handicaps (ICIDH), which was first published by WHO for trial purposes in 1980. After systematic field trials and international consultations, the classification was thoroughly revised and renamed ICF; it was endorsed for international use by the Fifty-fourth World Health Assembly in 2001. The ICF has been translated into some 38 languages and can be accessed online in Arabic, Chinese, English, French, Russian and Spanish at the WHO website (WHO, 2001b).

As described in the WHO overview (WHO, 2001b), the ICF has two parts, each with two components that describe health status and well-being.

Part 1. Functioning and disability
a) Body functions and structures
  i. Body functions are the physiological functions of body systems. These include mental functions, sensory functions, voice and speech functions, and functions of the cardiovascular, haematological, immunological and respiratory systems.
  ii. Body structures: are anatomical parts of the body such as organs, limbs, and their components. These include structures of the nervous system; eyes, ears, structures involved in voice and speech; structures of the cardiovascular, immunological and respiratory systems; digestive, metabolic, endocrine systems; structures related to the genitourinary and reproductive

systems; structures related to movement; skin and related structures.
b) Activities and participation. Activity is the execution of a task or action by an individual; participation is involvement in a life situation. Activities and participation include learning and applying knowledge, general tasks and demands (such as undertaking single or multiple tasks, carrying out a daily routine), communication, mobility, self-care, domestic life, interpersonal interactions and relationships, major life areas (such as education and work life), community, social and civic life.

Part 2. Contextual Factors
c) Environmental factors: make up the physical, social, and attitudinal environment in which people live and conduct their lives. These include products and technology (such as food, drugs, assistive products and technology); natural environment and human made changes to the environment; support and relationships; attitudes; service systems and policies.
d) Personal factors: such as temperament, personal lifestyles, beliefs, desires.

Within the ICF framework, impairments are problems in body function or structure, such as a significant deviation or loss. Activity limitations are difficulties that an individual may have in executing activities; participation restrictions are problems an individual may experience in involvement in life situations. The ICF framework is all-inclusive, non-stigmatizing and comprehensive. The ICF version for children and youth (ICF-CY) has recently been derived from the ICF (Lollar & Simeonsson, 2005; WHO, 2007).

Application of classification systems

The following clinical vignettes are provided to convey a better understanding of how the ICF, DC: 0-3R and ICD-10 classify developmental difficulties in young children.

Case A. Ayse is a six-month-old child with normal growth, physical health and age-appropriate developmental milestones. When going to work in the fields, her mother leaves her in the care of her 12-year old sister. The mother returns to breastfeed but then goes back to work. For safety reasons, Ayse is not allowed out of her crib and the children do not leave the house for 10 hours during the day. Ayse is not failing to thrive yet, but the family is becoming poorer and has limited access to food.

Using the ICD-10: Ayse is classified as having inadequate parental supervision and control (Chapter XXI).

Using the DC: 0-3R: Ayse does not have an axis I, II, III or V diagnosis. Within the psychosocial risk factors of axis IV, she has risk factors listed under: poverty, poor quality in early learning environment, and a caregiver without education.

Using the ICF: Ayse is classified as having no impairments in body functions and structures, but severe restrictions in activities and participation, and severe barriers in environmental factors, i.e. basic care by adult and adequate food.

Case B. Elif is a 12-month-old child hospitalized for severe malnutrition, iron-deficiency anaemia and zinc deficiency. The medical history reveals that Elif has been breastfed from the start. Her mother force fed her after she refused to take supplemental solid foods. Elif is refusing to eat, is apathetic and uninterested in play. Her mother approaches her with anxiety and becomes very tense during feeding.

Using the ICD-10: Elif is classified as having malnutrition and iron-deficiency anaemia and zinc deficiency.

Using the DC: 0-3R: Elif has an eating disorder in axis I; an anxious-tense relationship is classified in axis II; Elif's malnutrition and anaemia are under axis III; there are no risk factors in axis IV; Elif's inadequacies in symbolic play are classified in Axis V.

Using the ICF: Elif is classified as having impairments in body functions and structures, including malnutrition, anaemia and micronutrient deficiency. She is restricted in activities and participation because of her refusal to eat and her lack of interest in interactions and play. An environmental factor causing difficulty is the anxious and tense relationship of her mother. All these components require intervention.

Case C. Hakim is brought by his grandmother to a community-based rehabilitation centre. He is a 3-year-old child with spastic paraplegia due to prematurity and intracranial haemorrhage. He is unable to bear weight or crawl, but can sit up in his wheelchair. He uses his hands to play with a home-made rattle and can feed himself effectively with a spoon. Hakim uses two-word sentences to make his desires understood by his caregivers. He is often brought to the village play area where his siblings and other friends wheel him to participate in hide and seek and tag games.

Using the ICD-10: Hakim has spastic paraplegia.

Using the DC: 0-3R: Hakim does not have an axis I or axis II diagnosis. On axis III he has spastic paraplegia; on Axis IV he has a medical condition causing a stressor. Axis V is age appropriate.

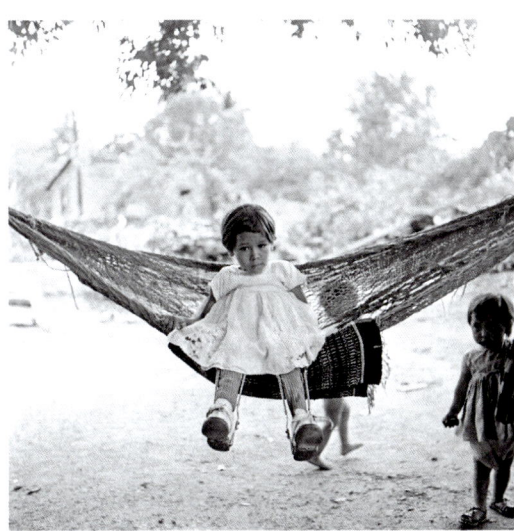

ICF-CY emphasizes activities and participation: child with polio in play, Mexico. © UNICEF/NYHQ1960-0008

Using the ICF: Hakim is classified as having impairments in neuromusculoskeletal and movement-related body functions (impairment in lower half of body muscle power and tone due to paraplegia) and impairment in central nervous system body structures, due to intracranial haemorrhage. He has complete difficulty in activities without caregiver and wheelchair assistance, because he is unable to crawl or walk; other areas of developmental activity are unaffected. He has mild difficulty in participating in play, because he is often encouraged to participate by his caregivers, siblings, and others in the community. The environment does not present barriers, as he has access to caregivers who promote his physical and mental health, development and learning. They provide access to CBR, which is present in the community, and he has technological assistance in the form of a wheelchair.

Strengths of the classification systems and areas that require improvement

As can be seen from the above examples, each classification system offers a different approach to classifying young children with developmental difficulties. Table 4 summarizes aspects of child development within the bioecological model and shows how each system addresses these aspects. The functions related to the child have been conceptualized as physical health, mental health, developmental status and participation. Contextual factors are caregiver–child relationships and the social environment.

The DC: 0-3 R has the advantage of having been developed specifically for mental health and developmental disorders of young children. A crucial concept in child development, caregiver–child relationships, can be coded explicitly in axis II. DC: 0-3 R recommends that ICD codes be used for the area of physical health in axis III. The developmental functioning of the child is also coded in axis III. This axis requires more development, however. Apart from mental disorders and social and emotional functioning, the developmental functioning, strengths and vulnerabilities of children cannot be explicitly coded.

The ICD is a disease-oriented categorical system, which is more practical and requires less training than the other systems. The ICD has codes within Chapter XXI that can be expanded to include participation, caregiver–child relationships and the social environment. The ICD, however, does not capture all the clinical information that is necessary to define and classify developmental difficulties. Furthermore, healthy developmental functioning cannot be classified using the ICD system alone. Currently, researchers and advocates of the WHO classification systems are recommending that ICD codes should be used in conjunction with ICF in the classification of childhood health, disease, disability and functioning (Simeonnson, Scarborough & Hebbeler, 2006).

The major advantage of the ICF system is that it has been designed to be used internationally, for people of all cultures and all ages, with any spectrum of health, disease or disability, strength or difficulty. Furthermore, the ICF is in complete concordance with current theories of child development and bioecological theory.

There are many benefits of using the ICF system to classify developmental difficulties in young children. The first is that the ICF model of human functioning and disability reflects the interactive relationship between health conditions and contextual factors. As shown in Figure 5, similar to the bioecological model of child development, ICF incorporates the role of environmental factors. Furthermore, the ICF uses non-stigmatizing, strengths-based language.

Another key point is that the designation "disability" is considered by the ICF as an umbrella term, representing the dynamic interaction between person and environment (Msall, 2006). In contrast to the traditional view that disability resides within the person, the ICF view is that disability is a social construct, involving an interaction of the person with the community or society. Furthermore, in the ICF, participation is identified

Table 4. Classifications that can be used to assess the development of young children

Aspects of child development within the bioecological model		DC: 0-3R	ICD	ICF
Functions related to the child	Physical health	Recommends ICD codes to be coded in Axis III	All chapters, except V and XXI	Body functions and structures (e.g. haematological system functions)
	Mental health	Axis I	Chapter V, Mental and behavioural disorders	Body functions and structures (e.g. emotional functions)
	Developmental status	Requires improvement Axis I (mental health) Axis III (developmental delay) Axis V (social–emotional development)	Chapter V, Mental and behavioural disorders Chapter VI, Diseases of the nervous system Chapter XVIII, R62.0 Delayed milestone	Body functions and structures (e.g. cognitive functions) Activity and participation (e.g. acquiring language, changing basic body position)
	Participation	Not addressed	Requires improvement Some items of Chapter XXI, (Z55-Z65 Persons with potential health hazards related to socioeconomic and psychosocial circumstances) (e.g. problems related to education and literacy) may be considered to reflect some aspects of participation	Activity and participation
Contextual factors	Caregiver–child relationships	Axis II	Requires improvement Some items of Chapter XXI (e.g. Z62.0 Inadequate parental supervision, Z62.1 Parental overprotection) may be considered to reflect some aspects of caregiver–child relationships	Requires improvement One code (d760 parent–child relationships) in section Activity and Participation may be considered
	Social environment	Axis IV (psychosocial stressors)	Requires improvement Chapter XXI (Z00–Z99), Factors influencing health status and contact with health services, may be considered to reflect some aspects of the social environment	Environment

as an important outcome of health. This should enable a seamless flow from the identification, assessment and classification of a developmental difficulty during early childhood to improvement of functioning and participation.

Parallel to the bioecological model of child development, the ICF embodies contextual factors that may affect a person's health. The first of these is environmental factors, which may be physical, social, cultural, or institutional, and which include the availability, quality, expertise, and focus of intervention programmes. The second component is personal factors, such as sex, age, education, lifestyle, the personal interests and desires of children and their families. WHO has thus chosen a biopsychosocial approach to health, functioning, and disability in the new ICF model, to provide "a coherent view of different perspectives of health from a biological, individual and social perspective" (WHO, 2001b).

WHO is encouraging application of the ICF internationally, not only as a classification tool, but also as a framework for social policy, research, education, and clinical practice. Many aspects of the ICF are in congruence with the bioecological model of child development and it is therefore a

Figure 5. Underlying model of the WHO ICF

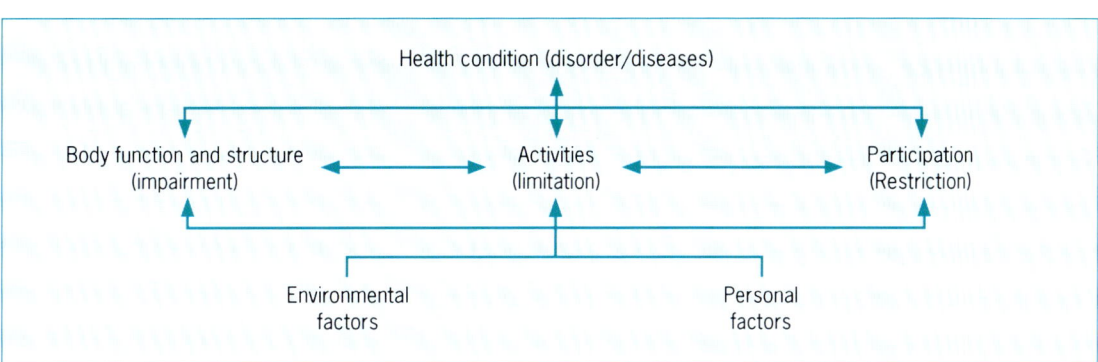

promising system for the classification of developmental difficulties.

The major difficulty in using the ICF is that it appears complicated and user-unfriendly, and requires intense study and training. Furthermore, the related system for children and youth, ICF-CY, deserves further development to include more detail on the interactions and relationships in the caregiving environment. A structure to explicitly record the strengths of the child, caregiving environment and the community would also be a benefit (Lollar & Simeonsson, 2005).

As was seen from the vignettes, ICF is unmatched as a classification system in the wealth of clinical information it captures, its flexibility and comprehensiveness, and the seamless transition to what is needed for the child in terms of reinforcement of personal and environmental strengths and interventions.

Research in LAMI countries

Research in LAMI countries on classification systems for young children with developmental difficulties is almost non-existent. One important WHO collaborative research study on ICD-10 included both children and adults. Data were collected in eight Arab countries on a total of 233 patients, using the local psychiatric interview schedules and diagnoses according to ICD-10 criteria. Inter-rater reliability was found to range between almost perfect agreement (0.81–1) to substantial agreement (0.61–0.80) (using the kappa coefficient) in diagnosing organic mental disorders, substance use disorders, schizophrenic, schizotypal and delusional disorders, affective disorders, and neurotic and stress-related disorders. The categories of psychological development and child and adolescent disorders were diagnosed less frequently and the agreement between raters was lower (Okasha & Seif el Dawla, 1992).

In a study in India, diagnostic criteria for autism were examined by 937 Indian psychiatrists, psychologists and paediatricians. Participants were asked to rate 18 types of behaviour as (a) necessary for a diagnosis of autism, (b) helpful but not necessary, or (c) not helpful in a diagnosis of autism, and were asked to provide other information about their experiences with autism. The study showed that Indian professionals were endorsing criteria for autism that were present in the DSM systems (Daley & Sigman, 2002).

No studies in LAMI countries using the ICF or DC: 0-3 systems for the classification of young children with developmental difficulties have been found.

Conclusions and implications

1. Internationally endorsed classifications are important in facilitating and advancing communication between clinicians, researchers and policy-makers, as well as in advancing clinical conceptualization, assessment and formulation.

2. Three widely used classification systems, ICD-10, DC:0-3R, and ICF, offer a promising approach to the classification of developmental difficulties in young children. All of these systems have conceptual or pragmatic aspects that are particularly useful for the classification of developmental difficulties in young children. All the systems also have aspects that pose difficulties in their widespread application. The DC: 0-3R offers a closer focus on the caregiving relationship, but the concept of developmental difficulties has not been expanded beyond mental health disorders. ICD-10 is a pragmatic categorical approach; some codes include some of the environmental and contextual aspects of

child development and the classification could potentially be improved to include more specific aspects of early childhood development. ICD codes can be used in conjuction with either of the other two systems. The ICF system offers an approach that is in concordance with theories of child development and current concepts in developmental interventions. The caregiver–child relationship component requires improvement. Axis II codes of the DC: 0-3R could potentially be used to improve this area.

3. A task force is needed to review the potential of the existing systems for the classification of the functional development and developmental difficulties of young children.

4. Research is greatly needed in LAMI countries on classification systems. Such research should aim to identify how classification systems can be widely used in resource-poor situations, so that meaningful information on the status of children and interventions to improve their situation can be shared.

Chapter

Early intervention

DDEC Survey results

The DDEC Survey requested information about a number of issues related to early intervention (EI) for young children with developmental risks and difficulties. Only 12 countries had a law guaranteeing access to early intervention services for young children with developmental difficulties: France, Israel, Saudi Arabia, the United Kingdom and the United States (high-income countries); and Bulgaria, Ecuador, Jordan, Lebanon, Kyrgyzstan, Turkey and Viet Nam (low- and middle-income countries). The laws dated from as early as 1975 (France) to as late as 2005 (Kyrgyzstan).

The vast majority of countries had EI services; in some cases, these were widespread, but most existed only in large cities or as isolated projects. Home-based EI was available in only three countries. In approximately half of the countries, most EI clinicians had had university or college level training in early intervention or a related discipline. Five countries (all LAMI) had no training courses for EI professionals. In the vast majority of countries, EI services were centre-based. In approximately half of the countries, families were not present during most EI sessions; in more than half, EI services were child-centred (caregivers were informed but professionals mainly focused on improving the skills of the child) rather than family-centred (clinicians viewed caregivers as active partners and obtained their input into services). Most countries had no residential centres for young children; where such centres existed, they accommodated only a small minority of children with developmental difficulties.

In most countries, EI services (as listed in question 23, see Annex 1) were generally not available to the majority of children with developmental difficulties. The only service that was available to most children in the majority of countries was orthopaedic treatment. The following services were least likely to be available: psychological counselling, EI for difficulties in caregiver–child relationship, and EI for social and emotional difficulties. In most countries, government funded most EI services (question 23), and was the major source of funding for EI in more than half of the countries, followed by non-profit organizations in six countries (question 24). In the vast majority of countries, maternal and paternal education, caregiver income, geographical location of the family, and urban versus rural residence had an impact on whether the child received EI services. In 70% of the countries, stigmatization had an impact. Religion and ethnicity had an impact on receiving EI services in less than half of the countries.

Purpose and scope of the chapter and additional key resources

The scope of this chapter is limited to a summary of current conceptualizations of early intervention, examples of published research on this topic from LAMI countries, and an example of a model early intervention programme linked to the health system. For more comprehensive information on EI, readers are referred to a number of seminal publications. Three books are of particular interest: *Handbook of early intervention*, edited by Shonkoff and Meisels (2000), *The effectiveness of early intervention*, by Guralnick (1997), and *The developmental systems approach to early intervention*, also by Guralnick (2005a). This last book has a chapter dealing specifically with the situation in developing countries (Rye & Hundeide, 2005). One book has been devoted to early intervention around the world (Odom et al., 2003), and has detailed descriptions of early intervention programmes in Brazil (Lumpkin & Aranha, 2003),

> "The majority of services in this country have adopted models from industrialized countries. While aspects of these models may be applicable locally, they are by and large not suitable to meet the vast needs of the disabled. Services for the disabled are currently fragmented, hospital-based and inadequate and do not appear to be a priority in medical development locally. Parents face many hindrances from service providers. Children with disability are often managed by a number of different departments with little integration. Services are better at assessment than rehabilitation. The chronic care for these children fatigues service providers and parents. There is a prevailing sense of hopelessness. Most services do not adequately address the emotional burden of the family. Hence there is a high "dropout" rate in the utilization of rehabilitative services by parents. The development of services for children with disability and their family is largely in the hands of professionals or therapists working in government agencies and nongovernmental organizations. This has often resulted in services that are developed to meet the needs of the professional, therapist or organization rather than those of the child or family. Children with disability and their parents need to be consulted and involved in the decision-making process of proposed and existing services which cater for their needs. We require the will to relinquish "control" and distance ourselves from the "politics" of disability. We need instead to see children with disability and their family as partners and offer them care in a way which dignifies, best meets the needs of the person with disability and takes into account his or her cultural and spiritual needs."
>
> *Dr Amar Singh, Senior Consultant Paediatrician, Head of Paediatric Department,*
> *Ipoh Hospital, Ipoh, Perak, Malaysia*

China (Tsai-Hsing Hsia, McCabe & Li, 2003), Egypt (Khouzam, Chenouda & Naguib, 2003), Ethiopia (Teferra, 2003), India (Kaul et al., 2003), and Jamaica (Thorburn, 2003). Another informative book is by Zinkin&McConachie (1995). A special issue of the *Journal of Policy and Practice in Intellectual Disabilities* was devoted to early intervention from an international perspective, with information from Europe, the United States and Israel (Guralnick, 2006a). A special report of the European Agency for Development in Special Needs Education (2005) provides information on early intervention in European countries.

Conceptualization

Early intervention has been defined as a systematic and planned effort to promote development through a series of manipulations of environmental or experiential factors, initiated during the first five years of life. As defined by Shonkoff & Meisels (1990), EI consists of "multidiciplinary services provided for developmentally vulnerable children from birth to age 3 years and their families". In general, EI services are designed to meet the developmental needs of children, from birth to three or five years of age, who have a delay in physical, cognitive, communicative, social, emotional or adaptive development or have a diagnosed condition that has a high probability of resulting in developmental delay.

EI services can be conceptualized as primary, secondary and tertiary level interventions.

a) The primary prevention level aims to reduce the occurrence of developmental difficulties, by reducing or removing risk factors, such as low birth weight, malnutrition, iron and vitamin deficiencies, perinatal asphyxia and home-based and unsafe deliveries, and by improving nurturing and stimulation within the family.

b) The secondary prevention level aims to reduce the extent of possible or manifested developmental difficulties and to shorten their duration. Early intervention programmes for low birth weight children or for children with malnutrition or infants at risk operate at this level.

c) At the tertiary prevention level, the aim is to prevent or reduce complications of developmental difficulties.

Interventions at the primary level, related to the prevention of developmental difficulties for all children were covered in Chapter 5.

In this chapter, early intervention will be described in terms of interventions that aim to:

- assess risk factors,
- prevent developmental difficulties in vulnerable children,
- prevent the progression of difficulties,
- ameliorate the effects of difficulties on child functioning , and
- address curable causes of developmental risks or difficulties detected in young children and their families.

The conceptual framework for early intervention has evolved in many different parts of the world and in different cultures from multiple sources, such as early childhood education, maternal and child health services, special education, and research on child development (Shonkoff & Meisels, 2000). While most of the research and legislative processes on EI have so far been conducted in high-income countries, the present conceptual framework can be considered universal and humanistic.

What are EI services?

Typically, whether they are delivered as home-based or centre-based services, early intervention services incorporate two components: services to the child and services to the family. Services that can be considered under the umbrella of EI are:

a) family-centred approaches, including diagnosis of health problems, needs assessment and development of an EI plan;

b) family education;

c) physical therapy;

d) orthoses and prosthetics;

e) nursing care services;

f) nutritional support;

g) psychological and psychiatric support and treatment for child and family;

h) special education;

i) occupational therapy;

j) audiological services;

k) speech and language therapy;

l) special care for visual and hearing impairment;

m) transportation services to EI;

n) coordination of care.

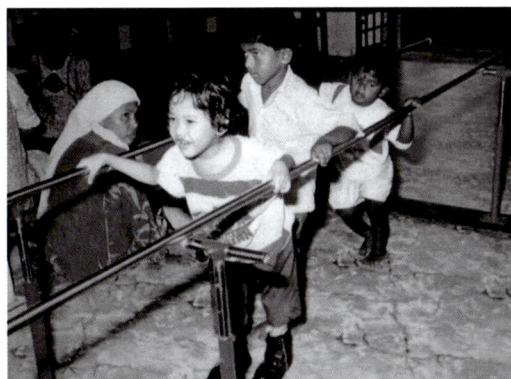

Community based rehabilitation services must be supported in all countries: children and caregivers at early intervention center, Malaysia. Photo: Dr. Amar-Singh

Who are EI services for?

EI has been made available for young children who have:

a) developmental risks, as a result of psychosocial factors, such as poverty or caregiver's mental health or substance abuse problems;

b) developmental risks due to biological factors, such as low birth weight, malnutrition, or prematurity;

c) established developmental difficulties, such as delays in language, cognitive, social–emotional or neuromotor functioning; this includes children with cerebral palsy, genetic syndromes, autism, cognitive difficulties, and hearing or visual impairment.

In high-income countries, early intervention is readily available for young children who are at risk due to poverty. Examples of nationwide programmes are Head Start (Zigler & Styfco, 2004) and Early Head Start in the United States (McAllister et al., 2005), and Sure Start (Belsky et al., 2006; Gray & Francis, 2007; Love et al., 2005; Tunstill et al., 2005) and Early Support (Young et al., 2008) in England. The eligibility criteria for entry into these programmes are determined by income status. A range of services are provided based on need, including nutritional support, health care access, play groups, quality day care or preschool groups. Caregivers benefit from support for parent–child interactions, parenting education, family planning services, literacy programmes, job training, physical and mental health programmes and community support programmes.

Research in high-income countries has shown that services for children who have biological risks are effective. The Infant Health and Development Program (IHDP) in the Unites States, for example, examined the impact of EI on the development of low birth weight premature infants (Berlin et al., 1998; Hill, Brooks-Gunn & Waldfogel, 2003; Klebanov & Brooks-Gunn, 2006; Ramey & Ramey, 1998). As a result of the IHDP, Birth to Three was founded in the USA as the national programme that ensures EI services for children with developmental risks.

An example of a national programme in a developing country that serves children with psychosocial risks is the Integrated Child Development Scheme (ICDS) in India. This programme was described in Chapter 2. Vazir et al. (1999) demonstrated that children benefiting from the ICDS achieved significantly higher scores for

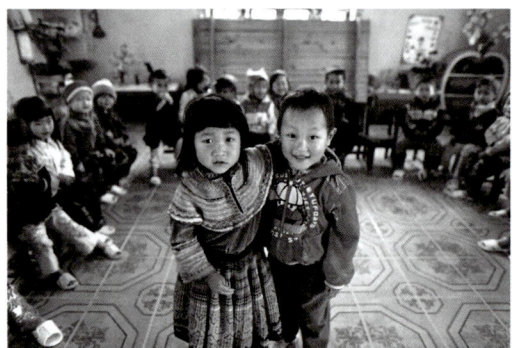
Child care centers, crèches must go beyond physical care and provide opportunities for early learning: children in preschool, Vietnam. © UNICEF/NYHQ2009-0234/ Estey

both motor and mental functioning at all ages than children who were not benefiting from the programme.

Although early intervention programmes for newborns discharged from neonatal intensive care units have been reported from countries such as South Africa (Lubbe, 2005) and India (DeSouza et al., 2000, 2006), there are no national programmes in LAMI countries that enable all children with developmental risks, such as prematurity, to benefit from EI services. Turkey is an example of a country that has a national government-funded system that provides physical therapy and special education for children of all ages with a developmental difficulty. However, support for children at risk for developmental difficulties is not included in this program.

What major improvements are needed in the conceptualization of EI?

There have been major improvements in the conceptualization of early intervention programmes in the past 30 years. Five major changes that are relevant for LAMI countries are summarized below.

1. A shift from the deficit model to the empowerment model

The deficit model in early intervention originated from the biomedical model in health care. In this model, the child's developmental difficulties and delays are determined by professionals, and EI aims to address these deficits. Deficits in family functioning are also determined and addressed. Clinicians working with children and families for some time can recognize the limitations of this model. Children and families often do not solve problems based on what professionals tell them, but by using their own strengths, creativity and problem-solving skills. Furthermore, clinicians working within the deficit model may find that they are repeating themselves and focusing on basic rote skills, which may not be particularly functional for the children and their families. Within the deficit model, clinicians may have difficulties in recognizing the true strengths, values and aspirations of children and families. The empowerment model evolved from families' feelings of disempowerment within the deficit model. The resulting model is based on working with children and families to support them in EI, to recognize their aspirations and goals, and to help them find and mobilize their multiple strengths, resources and creativity to improve their child's development. Developers of new EI programmes should recognize that the theory of EI and the training of EI clinicians have shifted from the deficit model to the empowerment model as the gold standard approach.

2. A shift from the child-centred to the family-centred model

Although families have always been a part of EI programmes, in the past their role was mostly passive. EI professionals would often decide what the child and family needed and tell them what they should do. In recent years, families – regardless of their educational and socioeconomic background – have increasingly been recognized as key, active, equal partners in the EI process. Caregivers are expected and encouraged to examine their child's strengths and needs and, with clinician support, to develop a programme of EI that will meet their own and their child's goals and aspirations.

3. A shift from a fragmented model to a one-stop comprehensive model

In EI, the needs of children and families and the services provided may be multifaceted, but the child and family do not necessarily benefit from the fragmentation. When clinicians providing cognitive stimulation, speech and language therapy, physical therapy, health care and family support work with the child and family separately, there may be lack of continuity, congruence, and convergence between the services. One particular barrier is the provision of different services in different centres. Maximal links between clinicians and the provision of all or most services within the home are components of a more effective "one-stop" comprehensive or holistic model (Lequerica, 1997).

4. A shift from an early childhood approach to a life-cycle approach

Previously, many EI programmes began and ended in the early years of life. Currently, it is recognized that interventions that aim to enhance child development, particularly for children at risk or with developmental difficulties, must allow a smooth transition to potentially lifelong programmes.

5. A shift from neglecting cultural diversity to endorsing it

Many EI programmes have been modelled on programmes that originated and were tested in developed countries. Regardless of adaptations in the content, these programmes largely carried Western cultural influences (Sturmey et al., 1992). In recent years, largely as a result of work with immigrant and minority populations in developed countries, a deeper understanding has evolved of the effects of culture on child upbringing, and on the perceptions of children and families. The value of cultural diversity and its positive influences on children have received more recognition than in the past (Garcia Coll & Magnuson, 2000; Louw & Avenant, 2002). Understanding the strengths, innovations, novelties, challenges and solutions of the culture in which EI is taking place – in other words, endorsing cultural diversity to work for EI – is a component of best practice in EI.

Evidence-based best practices in early intervention

Key features of early intervention programmes have been evaluated for almost half a century in high-income countries (Shonkoff & Meisels, 2000). Such evaluations have shown that, for policies and programmes to be effective, attention has to be given to the specific needs of children and families in a variety of circumstances. A wide range of programmes have achieved positive results, including child-focused, parent-focused, and two-generation models that function in a variety of settings, such as homes and community centres. Successful programmes apply key concepts of child development in addressing the needs of children and families. Specifically, successful programmes identify family stressors and needs (e.g. informational needs, mental health issues, interpersonal and family distress). Programmes then employ highly individualized approaches to improve family and child competencies by addressing resource supports, social supports and information, and by providing specific services. Regardless of the focus of the program, this is accomplished by family-centred practices that ensure that the programme is consistent with the family's goals, values, priorities and routines (Guralnick, 2005a, 2005b, 2006b).

Some effective programmes have involved intensive home-visiting by specialized nurses or highly trained practitioners, skilled counselling of parents for mental health problems, or a mixture of intensive home-visiting for parents and high-quality centre-based services for children (Gilliam et al., 2000; Olds, 2007; US Department of Health and Human Services, 2002). Research in high-income countries has highlighted that skilled staff are needed for the administration of early intervention programmes, especially for the families with the greatest challenges (Olds, 2007). Parallel to the identification of the importance of social and emotional development in cognitive and adaptive development in later years, particular attention is directed to programmes that address the emotional and social needs of young children and families with skilled staff. Effective screening and referral processes need to be in place. Screening may be carried out in primary physician offices, child care facilities, and preschool facilities. It has been highlighted that all screening, assessment, and intervention efforts should address the language and cultural characteristics of the children and families.

In general, programmes that begin early, that target families and children, and that are intensive and structured are most successful (Shonkoff & Hauser-Cram, 1987). A key feature of early childhood intervention is the "transdisciplinary model", in which professionals' roles are not fixed. Clinicians discuss and work together on goals, even when these are outside their discipline. The boundaries between disciplines are deliberately blurred to allow a family-centred approach and flexibility.

> In general, programmes that begin early, that target families and children, and that are intensive and structured are most successful.

Summary of research in LAMI countries

There have been a number of research studies in LAMI countries that have shed light on our understanding of EI.

1. The empowerment model

No examples of research in LAMI countries on the empowerment model in comparison with the deficit model could be found.

2. The family-centred model

A number of studies have highlighted the need for a family-centred model of EI. In particular, many studies have underscored the importance of addressing the burden on caregivers of children with developmental difficulties. Research in high-income countries has demonstrated compromises in the functioning of caregivers of children with developmental difficulties (Melnyk et al., 2004; Raina et al., 2005). Research in LAMI countries has also shown that caregivers experience increased stress when caring for a child with a developmental difficulty.

A study in Bangladesh showed that, in mothers of young children with cerebral palsy, the strongest predictor of maternal stress was child behavioural problems, especially those related to caring (Mobarek et al., 2000). An alarming proportion of mothers (42%) were found to be at high risk of psychiatric morbidity.

Ong and colleagues studied coping and stress experienced by Malaysian mothers who had children with cerebral palsy (Ong et al., 1998), mental retardation (Ong, Chandran & Peng, 1999) or very low birth weight (VLBW) (Ong, Chandran & Boo, 2001). These studies shed light on the fact that different types of interventions may be needed to alleviate stress in different risk populations.

In the study on children with VLBW, specific child characteristics (such as being male, having a low IQ score and presence of behavioural problems) and maternal factors (such as low education and being the primary caregiver) appeared to have a greater impact on parenting stress than the biological risk of VLBW birth.

The study on children with cerebral palsy showed that mothers of those children scored significantly higher than control subjects on the Parenting Stress Index (PSI). The impact of cerebral palsy on parenting stress was modified by other factors, such as increased caregiving demands, low maternal education, children's admission to hospital and Chinese ethnic background.

When compared with controls, mothers of children with mental retardation were also found to have increased levels of parenting stress. PSI scores in this study were affected by child behavioural problems, maternal unemployment and Chinese ethnicity.

The need for rehabilitation to be directed at "easing the burden of daily care, childhood behavior problems, minimizing hospital re-admissions and targeting appropriate psychosocial support at specific subgroups to address parental perceptions and expectations that may lead to increased stress" was highlighted (Ong et al., 1998).

3. The need for a comprehensive one-stop model

The need for comprehensive EI programmes that address all components of the health and development of young children is well recognized.

There have been a few research studies in LAMI countries that have demonstrated the crucial need for such a comprehensive model. Two studies highlighted the need for integrated health services and EI. The first examined mortality in children with developmental difficulties and highlighted the importance of addressing the health and nutrition of children with developmental difficulties. The study followed 92 children with cerebral palsy in Bangladesh for up to 3 years. Eight children died: two of 49 (4%) in an urban area and six of 43 (14%) in a rural area. Factors such as infections and drug reactions preceded all the deaths; those who died were mostly severely malnourished and among the more severely disabled (Khan et al., 1998). A study in India showed how the basic medical needs of the children may be neglected if services are not incorporated. This study aimed to determine the need for ophthalmological services for children with coloboma, microphthalmos and microcornea; it showed that many children who were enrolled in special schools for the blind could have benefited from simple ophthalmological interventions, such as spectacles and low vision aids (Hornby et al., 2000).

Two other studies highlighted the need for interventions to address all aspects of development and functioning. A study in rural India reported on reduced participation in social activities of children with epilepsy (Pal et al., 2002). At all ages from 2 to 18 years, boys and girls with epilepsy had limited peer group activities. The lack of participation could not be explained by the constraints imposed by the impairment itself. Of particular interest was that preschool-age children were more protected than their peers and had significantly less active social lives. In Thailand, a tertiary centre-based study on children with Down syndrome found that most children (66%) had received early stimulation, but that only 39% had attended a speech intervention programme in the first two years of life (Jaruratanasirikul et al., 2004). Language skills in most of the children were found to be limited.

Understanding the reasons for compliance and non-compliance with EI services is one of the most crucial components of service delivery. The one-stop model, which seeks to increase uptake, compliance and effectiveness of EI, has not yet been fully achieved, even in high-income countries. In LAMI countries, the need for one-stop, easily accessible services may be even more important. A number of longitudinal studies have been conducted on compliance with EI services. A study in Bangladesh examined the factors that affect mothers' attendance at specific EI services (McConachie et al., 2001). The Bangladesh Protibondhi Foundation developed an outreach parent training service based at two centres, one urban and one rural. At these centres, mothers were shown how to use picture-based distance training packages, which they could take home. The study followed 47 children with cerebral palsy, aged 2–5.5 years. Compliance with the programme was low. The main factors predicting higher attendance were male sex of the child, particularly in the rural area, and higher level of problems mothers' adapting to the child. The problems described by the mothers in using the advisory service were economic (such as transport costs), cultural (such as mothers not being permitted to go out alone), and medical (such as the child having repeated convulsions).

In a study on compliance with EI services in Goa, India, 360 newborns at high risk for developmental difficulties were offered a centre-based EI programme (DeSouza et al., 2000). Most families (54%) failed to bring their children for their follow-up appointments, 67% dropped out within the first 3 months, 19% between 4 and 6 months, 10% between 7 and 9 months and 4% after 9 months of follow-up. The only sociodemographic parameter that demonstrated a strong linkage with follow-up was parental education. Both the mother's and the father's education were important and, after adjustment, higher paternal education was more strongly associated with better follow-up rates. This study highlighted the importance of convincing poorly educated fathers of the benefits of early intervention.

Another component of the study in Goa highlighted the need for home-based EI programmes for high-risk children. In this study, 158 high-risk neonates and their parents were offered a clinic-based early intervention programme and were followed until their first birthday. Sociodemographic, programmatic and infant-related variables that could influence compliance and uptake of the programme were investigated. Only 59% of the infants were brought for three or more sessions. Higher maternal educational levels and proximity of place of residence to the clinic were significantly associated with better compliance (DeSouza et al., 2006).

In a randomized controlled trial in Bangladesh, McConachie et al. (2000) examined the efficacy of an outreach programme for young children with cerebral palsy. The study had two arms, both for the urban children (a centre-based mother–child group versus outreach parent training) and for the rural children (outreach parent training versus health advice only). The mother–child groups were organized daily by clinicians with training in physiotherapy. The distance training packages were given to families after an initial 1–2 hours of practice with the child. Though hampered by a small sample size and variability in the intensity of the intervention, the results suggested that distance training packages and mothers' groups hold promise for helping mothers improve the skills of their young children with cerebral palsy.

4. Addressing continuity of services across the lifespan

No research in LAMI countries related to continuity of service delivery could be found.

5. Addressing cultural diversity

Cultural aspects shape the content, delivery and evaluation of the EI programme. The content of EI will depend largely on the starting-point of what caregivers believe, know and can do with their children. This may be different for different populations. For example, in a population-

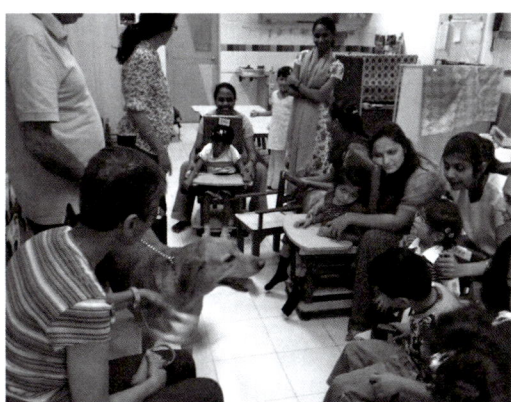

Early intervention services must partner with families and include participation in daily life activities: children and parents in early intervention center, India.
Photo: Dr. Vibha Krishnamurthy

based study in two cities in Turkey, it was found that most mothers of children aged 0–3 years believed that most developmental skills and activities should occur at later than normative ages (Ertem et al., 2007). Of the 1055 mothers, 52% did not know the ages at which children typically acquire vision. A higher proportion of mothers – 79%, 59% and 68% respectively – did not know that vocalization, social smiling and overall brain development begin in the early months of life. Interventions to improve maternal knowledge would need to be geared to such basic information before moving to more sophisticated levels of development.

Cultural aspects may also play a role in the delivery and uptake of interventions. The cultural role of fathers has been highlighted previously (DeSouza et al., 2000). The extended family also plays an important role in the lives of children in LAMI countries but this has not been fully studied. In Uganda, a study with a qualitative phenomenological design looked at how family members coped with their disabled children (Hartley et al., 2005). Data were collected from 52 families with children with disabilities from five impairment groups, through interviews and observations in one urban and two rural districts. Findings showed that most children with disabilities were included within the families, and were loved and cared for. Families spent considerable time and money on seeking a cure. With the breakdown of extended family systems, the main burden of caring for a disabled child generally fell on one or two female caregivers. Male members acted as gatekeepers, making the key decisions related to the child and the associated resources. In this cultural context, the authors drew conclusions that were pertinent and transferable to other settings: interventions "should move the focus of their services away from the disabled individual towards the whole family. It is important to provide accurate information about causes and prevention of impairments, the realities of a cure, support and respite for the female caregivers, and opportunities for the involvement of fathers."

The culture of the community in relation to stigma is also important. In LAMI countries, caregivers of children with developmental difficulties may experience more stigmatization and less support from society and legislation than those in high-income countries. A study in Lebanon examined feelings of stigmatization, isolation and stress, and depressive symptoms, in mothers of children with mental retardation (Azar & Badr, 2006). Stigmatization and isolation appear to be common concepts everywhere. Bridge (2004) reported on a series of observation visits to self-help groups established by parents for their disabled children in Ukraine. In that country, parents of disabled children were encouraged to place their child in institutional care. There were strict legal regulations excluding the children from normal schools and medical assessments were the basis for decisions about child care. Nevertheless, many parents decided to care for their disabled child at home within the family. Bridge drew attention to the emotional stress experienced by both parents and their disabled children in coming to terms with the conditions and denial of the normal rights of childhood resulting from prejudice, poor resources, ignorance, and restrictive legislation. Despite such difficulties, there is also a success story from Ukraine, showing that when the principles of EI are endorsed, improvements can be rapid and effective. A detailed report by Kukuruza (1998) demonstrated a major improvement in community EI models.

Further research is needed on the importance of acknowledging the complexities of working on EI in diverse communities with their unique cultural, religious, social and economic conditions (Crishna, 1999).

Important questions for future research

Research on EI in LAMI countries is still in its early stages. With appropriate stimulation and support, including building of infrastructure, appropriate funding and careful thought about the components of EI that need to be addressed, this field should grow and develop rapidly. Many questions need to be answered. Three important questions are:

1. Are there EI programmes that have been shown to be effective (such as the IHDP) that can be adapted and delivered in other countries with diverse settings?

2. What is the level of intensity that the EI programme needs to show a clinically important and sustainable effect?

3. How can collaborations between researchers and communities from different countries be built, so that research goals, ideas, strategies, results and implications related to EI can be shared to ensure progress in LAMI countries?

One ongoing research project that aims to address each of these research questions is being conducted at the University of Birmingham,

Alabama, USA. A cluster randomized controlled trial of a home-based intervention is under way in India, Pakistan and Zambia. This study identifies infants with birth asphyxia and others at risk for neurodevelopmental disorders and evaluates the outcomes of an innovative home-based, parent-provided, early intervention programme (Carlo, 2007). The study has two other important components: it aims to determine the level of intensity needed for the interventions to have a positive and sustained effect; and to broaden research collaboration between countries, to build sustainable capacity for research on early intervention and neurodevelopmental outcomes. This study shows that it is possible to address important questions, design the methodology to answer them collaboratively and bring real benefits to children around the world.

An exemplary model from LAMI countries

In this section, rather than provide details of a single intervention programme, a summary will be given of the WHO community-based rehabilitation (CBR) model, together with examples of country programmes that have employed this model. The WHO introduced CBR in the 1980s as a strategy for improving the quality of life of disabled people and their families around the world (Helander, Mendis & Nelson, 1980, 1989). By definition, CBR aims to move away from centre-based, institution-based or specialist-based care towards the building of local knowledge and practices to address the special needs of people with disabilities within the community. Since its introduction, CBR has been widely applied in many parts of the world for people of all age groups. CBR has also been used as an EI strategy for young children with developmental difficulties and their caregivers.

As defined by WHO: "Community-based rehabilitation currently in practice in more than 90 countries around the world is a comprehensive strategy for involving people with disabilities in the development of their communities." CBR seeks to ensure that people with disabilities have equal access to rehabilitation and other services and opportunities – health, education and income – as do all other members of society. The target populations are people with disabilities, families of people with disabilities, communities, disabled people's organizations, local, regional and national governments, international organizations, nongovernmental organizations, medical and other professionals, business and industry (private sector). A wide range of activities is included, beyond medical care and rehabilitation, such as promoting positive attitudes towards people with disabilities, preventing the causes of disabilities, providing rehabilitation services, facilitating education and training opportunities, supporting local initiatives, monitoring and evaluating programmes, supporting micro and macro income-generation opportunities. WHO supports Member States in the following areas:

1. developing guidelines for CBR;
2. conducting regional and country workshops to promote CBR and the WHO guidelines;
3. initiating and/or strengthening CBR programmes.

Although CBR has been promoted by WHO in many countries for more than 30 years, research on its benefits has been fragmented. Finkenflügel, Wolffers & Huijsman (2005) reviewed 128 articles published between 1978 and 2002 to assess the evidence base for CBR. The review showed an ever-increasing number of publications on CBR. Theoretical papers and descriptive studies were most common; intervention studies and case reports were relatively rare. No systematic methodological review has yet been carried out, although reviews on specific aspects of CBR are available. The key aspects of implementation and stakeholders were relatively well presented, but the numbers of articles on participation and use of local resources were low. This study revealed that there has been no real focus of research in CBR and that the evidence base for CBR is fragmented and incoherent in almost all aspects. In order to establish evidence-based practices in CBR, systematic research needs to be conducted as well as comprehensive review studies on key aspects.

Despite the fragmented nature of the research on CBR, this model holds promise as an EI approach to developmental difficulties in young children. The envisioned CBR matrix is shown in Figure 6. The CBR matrix shows the different sectors that comprise the CBR approach. The five components of the matrix are health, education, livelihood, social and empowerment. The elements under the components offer tangible ways of working with persons with disability and their families. WHO has developed a variety of training materials for community rehabilitation workers who may provide services to young children. The following materials related to children can be found on the WHO website (http://www.who.int/disabilities/publications/care/en/):

- *Disability prevention and rehabilitation: a guide for strengthening the basic nursing curriculum* (1996);
- *Let's communicate: a handbook for people working with children with communication difficulties* (1997);
- *Promoting the development of infants and young children with spina bifida and hydrocephalus: a guide for mid-level rehabilitation workers* (1996);
- *Promoting the development of young children with cerebral palsy: a guide for mid-level rehabilitation workers* (1993);
- *Guidelines for the prevention of deformities in polio* (1990);

Additional EI training videos for CBR workers have been developed for use in Africa (e.g. Botswana, Malawi, Uganda, Zimbabwe, Zambia), Asia (e.g. China, India, Malaysia, Sri Lanka) and South America (e.g. Guyana) by organizations such as UNESCO, Cheshire Homes International, and local CBR programmes such as the Guyana CBR Program (McConkey, 1995).

Many countries have used the CBR model to provide EI for young children with developmental difficulties and their families.

A study in north-east Thailand reported on the successful establishment of a community-based speech therapy model within the health care system for children with cleft lip or palate (Prathanee, Dechongkit & Manochiopinig, 2006).

Early studies of CBR for children published in the 1980s reported on EI programmes in rural Guyana (O'Toole & McConkey, 1998; O'Toole, 1989)

Penny et al. (2007) reported from Uganda on a successful programme that each year provided assistance to over 5000 children with motor impairment, including transport, rehabilitation, hostels, physiotherapy, orthopaedic surgery, and orthopaedic appliance technology.

Finkenflügel et al. (1996) conducted a qualitative study in Zimbabwe to examine the appreciation of CBR by caregivers of children with a disability. The findings showed a significant correlation between appreciation of CBR and attitude towards health services.

Based on the need for an indigenous programme suited to the cultural milieu and socioeconomic conditions of India, Indchem Research and Development Laboratory developed a computer-assisted programme to train caregivers of children aged 0–2 years with cognitive difficulties. The curriculum was developed by an interdisciplinary team of experts in the field. In the programme called *Upanayan* (To lead along),

Figure 6. WHO community-based rehabilitation matrix

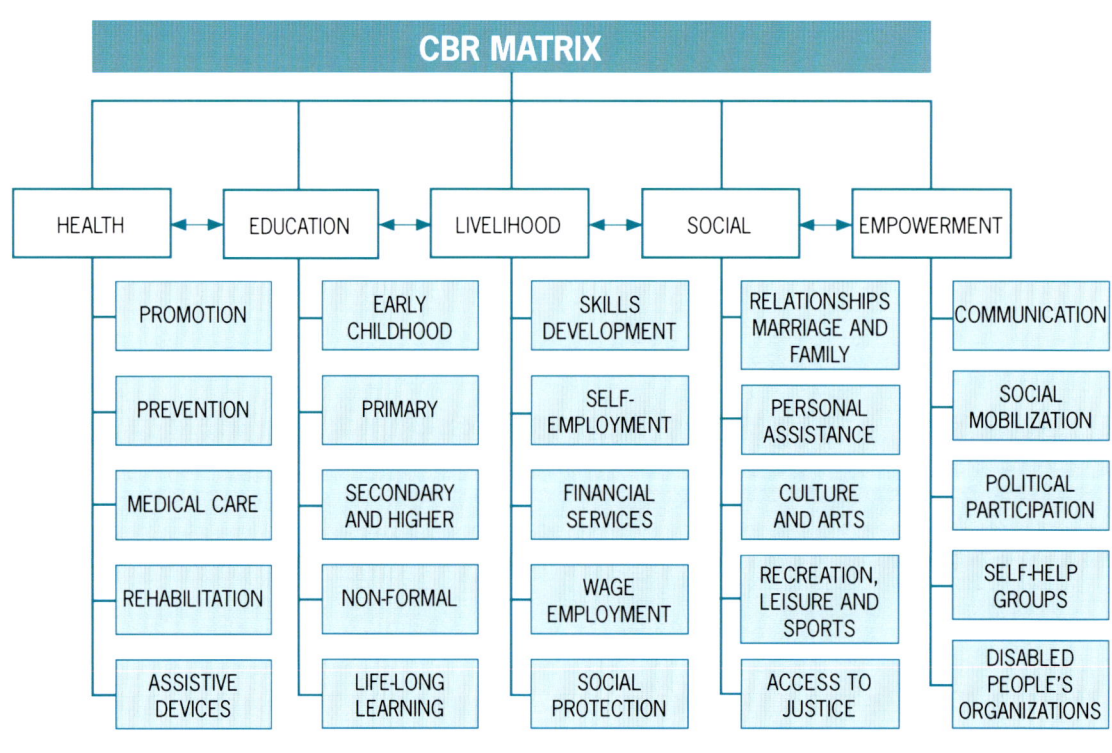

mothers are trained to support their children's development. A computer program for recording the data on the children and their progress facilitates the setting of goals and the monitoring of progress. Parents of children at Madhuram Narayanan Centre for Exceptional Children, Madras, use this programme for EI. The results of training have been encouraging (Krishnaswamy, 1992, 1994).

Conclusions and implications for action

1. There is important evidence from high-income countries that EI at the primary, secondary and tertiary levels is effective in preventing or reducing the burden of developmental difficulties for children, their families and the community.

2. Early intervention has evolved over the past century and is currently based on the following key principles:

   — The child is viewed in the context of the caregivers, family and larger community, and a family-centred, strengths- and function-based, empowering approach is favoured.

   — A one-stop comprehensive or holistic model is favoured over a fragmented approach, in which the child receives multiple services from different systems and service providers.

   — EI should not end when the child reaches a certain age, but should link seamlessly with services provided as needed throughout the life-cycle. Emphasis should be given to transition periods, when new circumstances and new needs may emerge.

3. EI is feasible in LAMI countries and years of experience have accumulated in many communities. Nevertheless, most children who are in need of EI in LAMI countries are not benefiting from EI programmes.

4. In LAMI countries, capacity needs to be built rapidly within health and other systems, so that EI services can be developed, implemented, and sustained. Such EI services should be evaluated so that evidence-based approaches can be integrated.

5. In most LAMI countries, despite their feasibility, EI services lag significantly behind those in high-income countries. Countries would benefit from international collaborative efforts, so that time and resources are not spent on reinventing what has already been shown to work (or not work).

Chapter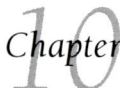

From prevention to intervention: consensus of experts

The DDEC Survey included an open-ended question asking respondents to describe three priority actions that they believed would improve services for young children with developmental difficulties in their country in the next five years. The answers to this question from the 31 respondents have been analysed using qualitative techniques. The following themes emerged from the responses:

- advancing policy related to developmental difficulties in early childhood at national level;
- bringing down barriers using common international approaches and platforms;
- increasing local capacity by training personnel;
- increasing capacity in other specialities related to developmental difficulties;
- empowering caregivers;
- conducting research.

Advancing policy related to developmental difficulties in early childhood at national levels

a) Advocacy efforts should concentrate on improving the understanding and commitment of policy-makers in all countries with respect to the importance of the early years, addressing the preventable causes of developmental difficulties, and improving early detection in conjunction with early intervention services.

b) Ministries of finance should fully understand that investment in early childhood may not pay off immediately, but is the most cost-beneficial and crucial step in the development of human capacity.

c) Legislation and national policies related to the promotion of child development and the early detection and management of developmental difficulties do not exist in most of the countries included in the DDEC Survey. Most of the respondents, particularly those from LAMI countries, considered that the key factor that would improve services for young children and their families would be the establishment of such policies and legislations, establishing services for the early detection of problems and management of children diagnosed as having a difficulty.

d) Legislation should be followed by improved access to services for all children. Barriers that have been identified by this survey, such as geographical location of residence, should be addressed.

e) Policy should also involve improved services addressing developmental difficulties at all levels (promotion of early childhood develooment, early detection and early intervention). Where services exist and can reach children and their families, they are usually subsidized by government. Respondents recommended that these services should be subsidized and free of charge in all countries.

f) Quality and affordable child care for children whose primary caregiver is employed in the workforce is an extremely important strategy in the prevention of developmental difficulties in infancy and early childhood.

g) Policies should be in place to develop national forums or platforms to discuss, monitor and review policies, plans and actions related to prevention of developmental difficulties and the promotion of optimal development for all children, specifically those with special needs.

h) Special centres that address the multitude of needs of young children with developmental difficulties and their families should be created. In these centres, services should be provided to meet both the biomedical and psychosocial needs of the child and family. Lengthy backlogs at such centres – a problem that has been encountered in high-income countries – should be avoided.

i) Primary health facilities may have special teams of staff who conduct home visits to prevent and detect developmental difficulties.

j) Posts should be created to ensure a full range of staff in ministries, such as those of health, education and social welfare.

k) Developmental–behavioural paediatrics should be promoted in LAMI countries. This field endorses the science of child development and brings together both the somatic and psychosocial needs of young children and their families. This field is a core agent in translating the science of child development and early intervention into paediatric health care.

Bringing down barriers using common international approaches and platforms

a) Respondents identified a need for guidance from a world body to foster a common understanding of the causes, identification and management of developmental difficulties.

b) Stigmatization should be addressed universally, regardless of the socioeconomic status of the country. It was stated, for example, that in some European countries where psychoanalytical approaches to developmental problems are dominant, caregivers may be viewed as the cause of some developmental difficulties, such as autism. In other countries, stigmatization may be present in other forms.

c) In most countries, families are not active partners in the early intervention process. Family-centred early intervention should be the cornerstone for care in all countries.

d) Common international classification systems, such as the WHO International Classification of Functioning, Disability and Health, which provide nondiscriminatory, theoretically justified and evidence-based means of classifying developmental difficulties, should be adopted by all countries.

e) In some countries, rehabilitation of young children is still viewed in the same framework as adult rehabilitation. International guidance is needed to adapt community-based rehabilitation to young children and their families.

f) International guidance is also needed on methods of early detection that are well linked to early intervention. Screening for developmental difficulties alone may provide visibility for problems, but may not be ethical if not linked to appropriate interventions.

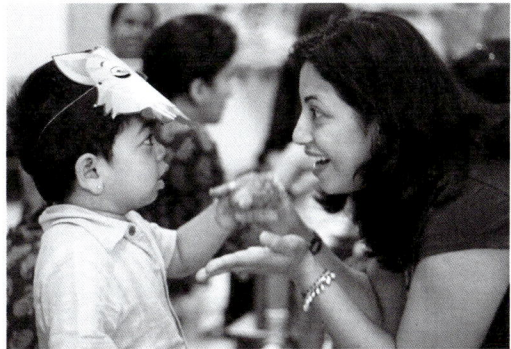

Centers that address the multitude of needs of children with difficulties and their families are needed: Child Development Center, India. Photo: Dr. Vibha Krishnamurthy

Increasing local capacity by training personnel

a) Training of primary health care providers. All respondents, regardless of country status, identified primary health care providers as the key human resource for delivering interventions related to early childhood development and developmental difficulties. All respondents underscored the importance of the training of health care providers.

— Preservice and in-service training should be provided for all health care providers (paediatricians, other doctors, nurses, midwives, other primary health care workers).

— Contemporary theories and models of early childhood development, with specific emphasis on caregiver relationships and the bioecological model, should be included.

— Health care providers are usually aware of gross motor development. Particular emphasis should be given to areas of functional development pertinent to later outcomes, i.e. language and communication, social–emotional development including relating, self-regulation, motivation, and cognitive development, such as problem-solving skills and attention.

— Causes of developmental difficulties, particularly in LAMI countries, should be emphasized; both biomedical and psychosocial causes across the life span should be included.

— Evidence-based interventions to prevent developmental difficulties should be reviewed.

— Health providers should gain the knowledge, skills and attitudes to empower caregivers to provide adequate and enriching developmental opportunities for their young children.

— Health providers should gain the skills to apply contemporary methods of early detection (screening and surveillance) for developmental difficulties during health encounters. These methods of detection should be directly linked to feasible interventions.

— The philosophy of early intervention and community-based rehabilitation should be a part of the training of health care personnel.

— Health care providers should also be equipped with knowledge of the role of other providers who work with children, and be skilled in working within interdisciplinary settings

Increasing capacity in other specialities related to developmental difficulties

Respondents from all countries recommended that human resources be increased in the fields that serve young children with developmental difficulties and their caregivers. Child development and early intervention specialists, child care providers, preschool teachers, psychologists, infant mental health specialists, educators, speech and language therapists, physiotherapists, occupational therapists, and audiologists are among the disciplines that need urgent strengthening, particularly in LAMI countries.

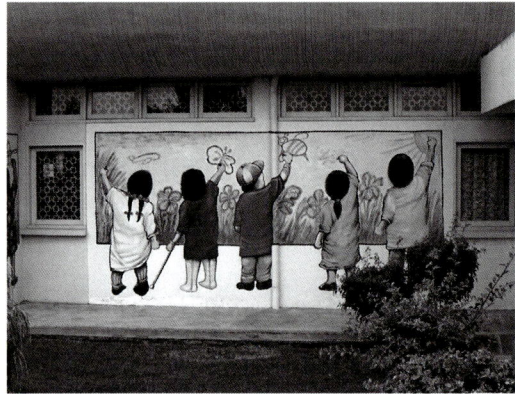

Center for Child Development, Malaysia.
Photo: Dr. Amar-Singh

Empowering caregivers

Policies and programmes should recognize the central role of caregiver involvement in early childhood. All efforts should be made to empower caregivers as partners in the prevention, diagnosis, assessment and management of developmental difficulties. Information can be given to caregivers by trained personnel, or through other available channels, such as the media. There is a wide gap between what caregivers know about the importance of early childhood in high-income and LAMI countries. Delivery of information and support to caregivers is urgently needed for all three phases of addressing developmental difficulties – prevention, early detection and management.

Conducting research

Research related to young children with developmental difficulties should be conducted through international collaborations, and with clear goals to determine what is needed and what works in LAMI countries.

Policies and programmes should recognize the central role of caregiver involvement in early childhood. All efforts should be made to empower caregivers as partners in the prevention, diagnosis, assessment and management of developmental difficulties. Information can be given to caregivers by trained personnel, or through other available channels, such as the media. There is a wide gap between what caregivers know about the importance of early childhood in high-income and LAMI countries. Delivery of information and support to caregivers is urgently needed for all three phases of addressing developmental difficulties – prevention, early detection and management.

References

Abidin RR (1983) Parenting stress and the utilization of pediatric services. *Child Health Care*. 11(2): 70–73.

Abiodun OA (1993) Emotional illness in a pediatric population in Nigeria. *J Trop Pediatr*. 39(1):49–51.

Aboud FE, Alemu T (1995) Nutrition, maternal responsiveness and mental development of Ethiopian children. *Soc Sci Med*. 41(5): 725–732.

Abu-Rabia S, Maroun L (2005) The effect of consanguineous marriage on reading disability in the Arab community. *Dyslexia*. 11(1):1–21.

Afzal M (1988) Consequences of consanguinity on cognitive behaviour. *Behaviour genetics*. 18:583–594.

Agarwal DK et al. (1992) Growth, behavior, development and intelligence in rural children between 1–3 years of life. *Indian Pediatr*. 29(4):467–480.

Agarwal P et al. (2005) Two-year neurodevelopmental outcome in children conceived by intracytoplasmic sperm injection: prospective cohort study. *BJOG*. 112(10): 1376–1383.

Aina OF, Morakinyo O (2005) Normative data on mental and motor development in Nigerian children. *West Afr J Med*. 24(2):151–156.

Aina OF, Morakinyo O (2001) The validation of Developmental Screening Inventory (DSI) on Nigerian children. *J Trop Pediatr*. 47(6):323–328.

Akaragian S, Dewa C (1992) Standardization of the Denver Developmental Screening Test for Armenian children. *J Pediatr Nurs*. 7(2):106–109.

Al-Hazmy MB, Al Sweilan B, Al-Moussa NB (2004) Handicap among children in Saudi Arabia: prevalence, distribution, type, determinants and related factors. *East Mediterr Health J*. 10(4–5):502–521.

al-Naquib N et al. (1999) The standardization of the Denver Developmental Screening Test on Arab children from the Middle East and north Africa. *J Med Liban*. 47(2):95–106.

Alpern G, Boll T, Shearer M (1986) *Developmental profile II (DP II)*. Los Angeles, Western Psychological Services, 1986.

Alpert JJ et al. (1976) Delivery of health care for children: report of an experiment. *Pediatrics*. 57(6):917–930.

American Psychiatric Association. (1994). *Diagnostic and statistical manual of mental disorders* (4th ed.). Washington, DC: Author.

American Psychiatric Association. (2000). *Diagnostic and statistical manual of mental disorders* (4th ed., text rev.) Washington, DC: Author.

Anderson FW et al. (2007) Maternal mortality and the consequences on infant and child survival in rural Haiti. *Matern Child Health J*. 11(4):395–401.

Andrade SA et al. (2005) Family environment and child's cognitive development: an epidemiological approach. *Rev Saude Publica*. 39(4): 606–611.

Angastiniotis MA, Hadjiminas MG (1981) Prevention of thalassaemia in Cyprus. *Lancet*. 1: 369–370.

Anselmi L et al. (2004) Psychosocial determinants of behaviour problems in Brazilian preschool children. *J Child Psychol Psychiatry*. 45(4):779–788.

Ari-Even Roth D et al. (2006) Low prevalence of hearing impairment among very low birthweight infants as detected by universal neonatal hearing screening. *Arch Dis Child Fetal Neonatal Ed*. 91(4):F257–262 (Epub 2006 Mar 10).

Aruna M, Vazir S, Vidyasagar P (2001) Child rearing and positive deviance in the development of preschoolers: a microanalysis. *Indian Pediatr*. 38(4):332–339.

Ashenafi Y et al. (2000) Socio-demographic correlates of mental and behavioural disorders of children in southern Ethiopia. *East Afr Med J*. 77(10):565–569.

Ashenafi Y et al. (2001) Prevalence of mental and behavioural disorders in Ethiopian children. *East Afr Med J*. 78(6):308–311.

Atasay B et al. (2003) Outcomes of very low birth weight infants in a newborn tertiary center in Turkey, 1997–2000. *Turk J Pediatr*. 45(4):283–289.

Au YL et al. (2004) Use of developmental language scales in Chinese children. *Brain Dev*. 26(2): 127–129.

Azar M, Badr LK (2006) The adaptation of mothers of children with intellectual disability in Lebanon. *J Transcult Nurs*. 17(4): 375–380.

Azra Haider B, Bhutta ZA (2006) Birth asphyxia in developing countries: current status and public health implications. *Curr Probl Pediatr Adolesc Health Care*. 36(5):178–188.

Badawi N et al. (1998) Intrapartum risk factors for newborn encephalopathy: the Western Australian case–control study. *BMJ*. 317(7172):1554–1558.

Baird G, Hall DM (1985) Developmental pediatrics in primary care: what should we teach? *Br Med J (Clin Res Ed)*. 291:583–586.

Bang AT, Bang RA & the SEARCH Team (1992) Diagnosis of causes of childhood deaths in developing countries by verbal autopsy suggested criteria. *Bull World Health Organ*. 70(4):499–507.

Barret RL, Robinson BE (1990) The role of adolescent fathers in parenting and childrearing. *Adv Adolesc Mental Health*. 4:189–200.

Barret T (2007) Nurses and mental health services in developing countries. *Lancet*. 370(9592):1016–1017.

Bashi J (1977) Effects of inbreeding on cognitive performance. *Nature*. 266:440–442.

Batshaw ML, ed. (2002) *Children with disabilities*, 5th ed. Baltimore. Paul H. Brookes Publishing Co.

Baydar N (1995) Consequences for children of their birth planning status. *Fam Plann Perspect*. 27(6):228–234.

Bayley N (1993) *Bayley Scales of Infant Development*, 2nd ed. San Antonio, The Psychological Corporation.

Bayley N (2006) *Bayley Scales of Infant Development*, 3rd ed. San Antonio, Hartcourt Assessment Publication.

Bear LM (2004) Early identification of infants at risk for developmental disabilities. *Pediatr Clin North Am*. 51(3):685–701.

Beard J (2007) Recent evidence from human and animal studies regarding iron status and infant development. *J Nutr*. 137(2):524S–530S.

Bella H, Al-Almaie SM (2005) Do children born before and after adequate birth intervals do better at school? *J Trop Pediatr*. 51(5):265–270.

Belsky J et al. (2006) Effects of Sure Start local programmes on children and families: early findings from a quasi-experimental, cross sectional study. *BMJ*. 332:1476–1748.

Ben Arab S, Bonaiti-Pellie C, Belkahia A (1990) An epidemiological and genetic study of congenital profound deafness in Tunisia (governorate of Nabeul). *J Med Genet*. 27(1): 29–33.

Bendel J et al. (1989) Prevalence of disabilities in a national sample of 3-year-old Israeli children. *Isr J Med Sci*. 25(5):264–270 .

Bender DE et al. (1994) Assessment of infant and early childhood development in a periurban Bolivian population. *Int J Rehabil Res*. 17(1): 75–81.

Benedict RE, Farel AM (2003) Identifying children in need of ancillary and enabling services: a population approach. *Soc Sci Med*. 57(11):2035–2047.

Berlin LJ et al. (1998) The effectiveness of early intervention: examining risk factors and pathways to enhanced development. *Prev Med*. 27(2):238–245.

Bethell C et al. (2004) Measuring the quality of preventive and developmental services for young children: national estimates and patterns of clinicians' performance. *Pediatrics*. 113 (suppl 6):S1973–S1983.

Bhargava A (2000) Modeling the effects of maternal nutritional status and socioeconomic variables on the anthropometric and psychological indicators of Kenyan infants from age 0–6 months. *Am J Phys Anthropol*. 111(1): 89–104.

Bhatia M, Joseph B (2000) Rehabilitation of cerebral palsy in a developing country: the need for comprehensive assessment. *Pediatr Rehabil*. 4:83–86.

Bhattacharjee H et al. (2008) Causes of childhood blindness in the northeastern states of India. *Indian J Ophthalmol*. 56:495–499.

Bhugra D, Minas IH (2007) Mental health and global movement of people. *Lancet*. 370(9593): 1109–1111.

Bhutta AT et al. (2002) Cognitive and behavioral outcomes of school-aged children who were born preterm: a meta-analysis. *JAMA*. 288 (6):728–737.

Black MM (2002) Society of pediatric psychology presidential address: opportunities for health promotion in primary care. *J Pediatr Psychol*. 27(7):637–646.

Black MM et al. (2002) Behavior problems among preschool children born to adolescent mothers: effects of maternal depression and perceptions of partner relationships. *J Clin Child Adolesc Psychol*. 31(1):16–26.

Black MM et al. (2007) Depressive symptoms among rural Bangladeshi mothers: implications for infant development. *J Child Psychol Psychiatry*. 48(8):764–772.

Black RE et al. (2008) Maternal and child undernutrition: global and regional exposures and health consequences. *Lancet*. 371(9608):243–260.

Blair M, Hall D (2006) From health surveillance to health promotion: the changing focus in preventive children's services. *Arch Dis Child*. 91:730–735.

Boo NY et al. (1996) Comparison of morbidities in very low birthweight and normal birthweight infants during the first year of life in a developing country. *J Paediatr Child Health*. 32(5):439–444.

Borghi E et al. (2000) Construction of the World Health Organization child growth standards: selection of methods for attained growth curves. *Stat Med.* 25(2):247–265.

Boris NW et al. (2000) Attachment and developmental psychopathology. *Psychiatry.* 63(1):75–84.

Borkowski JG et al. (1992) Unraveling the "new morbidity": adolescent parenting and developmental delays. *Int Rev Res Ment Retard.* 18:159–196.

Boulet SL, Boyle CA, Schieve LA (2009) Health care use and health and functional impact of developmental disabilities among US children, 1997–2005. *Arch Pediatr Adolesc Med.* 163(1):19–26.

Bowlby J (1978) Attachment theory and its therapeutic implications. *Adolesc Psychiatry.* 6:5–33.

Boyle CA, Decoufle P, Yeargin-Allsopp M (1994) Prevalence and health impact of developmental disabilities in US children. *Pediatrics.* 93:399–403.

Boyle D, Dwinnell B, Platt F (2005) Invite, listen, and summarize: a patient-centered communication technique. *Acad Med.* 80(1):29–32.

Bradley RH, Caldwell BM (1977) Home observation for measurement of the environment: a validation study of screening efficiency. *Am J Ment Defic.* 81(5):417–420.

Brazelton TB (1999) How to help parents of young children: the touchpoints model. *J Perinatol.* 19(6 Pt 2):S6-7.

Bricker D et al. (1995) *Ages & Stages Questionnaires (ASQ): a parent-completed, child-monitoring system*, 2nd ed. Baltimore; Brookes Publishing; 1995

Bridge G (2004) Disabled children and their families in Ukraine: health and mental health issues for families caring for their disabled child at home. *Soc Work Health Care.* 39(1–2): 89–105.

Briggs-Gowan M et al. (2000) Mental health in pediatric settings: distribution of disorders and factors related to service use. *J Am Acad Child Adolesc Psychiatry.* 39:841–849.

Bromiker R et al. (2004) Association of parental consanguinity with congenital malformations among Arab newborns in Jerusalem. *Clin Genet.* 66(1):63–66.

Bronfenbrenner U, Ceci SJ (1994) Nature-nurture reconceptualized in developmental perspective: a bioecological model. *Psychol Rev.* 101(4):568–586.

Brooks-Gunn J, Liaw FR, Klebanov PK (1992) Effects of early intervention on cognitive function of low birth weight preterm infants. *J Pediatr.* 120(3):350–359.

Brown N (1996) How should very low birth weight babies best be managed in Papua New Guinea? *PNG Med J.* 39(1):12–15.

Bundey S, Alam H (1993) A five-year prospective study of the health of children in different ethnic groups, with particular reference to the effect of inbreeding. *Eur J Hum Genet.* 1:206–219.

Buvinic M (1998) The costs of adolescent childbearing: evidence from Chile, Barbados, Guatemala, and Mexico. *Stud Fam Plann.* 29(2):201–209.

Campbell FA et al. (2002) Early childhood education: young adult outcomes from the Abecedarian Project. *Appl Dev Sci.* 6(1):42–57.

Campbell SB et al. (2004) The course of maternal depressive symptoms and maternal sensitivity as predictors of attachment security at 36 months. *Dev Psychopathol.* 16(2):231–252.

Carlo W (2007) Brain research to ameliorate impaired neurodevelopment – home-based intervention. United States National Institute of Child Health and Human Development (Grant number: 5R01HD053055-02).

Cassidy L, Jellinek M (1998) Approaches to recognition and management of childhood psychiatric disorders in pediatric primary care. *Pediatr Clin North Am.* 45:1037–1052.

Castillo-Durán C et al. (2001) Effect of zinc supplementation on development and growth of Chilean infants. *J Pediatr.* 138(2): 229–235.

Cervantes S, Raabe C (1991) Determinants of the evolution of the health situation of the population. *Scand J Soc Med Suppl.* 46:43–52.

Chamberlin RW, Szumowski EK, Zastowny TR (1979) An evaluation of efforts to educate mothers about child development in pediatric office practices. *Am J Public Health.* 69(9):875–886.

Chamberlin RW, Szumowski EK (1980) A follow-up study of parent education in pediatric office practices: impact at age two and a half. *Am J Public Health.* 70(11):1180–1188.

Chang SC et al. (2000) Mortality, morbidity, length and cost of hospitalization in very-low-birth-weight infants in the era of National Health Insurance in Taiwan: a medical center's experience. *Acta Paediatr Taiwan.* 41(6):308–312.

Chaudhari S (1996) Developmental assessment tests: scope and limitations. *Indian Pediatrics.* 33:541–545.

Chaudhari S et al. (1990) A longitudinal follow up of neurodevelopment of high risk newborns – a comparison of Amiel-Tison's method with Bayley Scales of Infant Development. *Indian Pediatr.* 27(8): 799–802.

Chaudhari S et al. (1995) Ultrasonography of the brain in preterm infants and its correlation with neurodevelopmental outcome. *Indian Pediatr.* 32(7):735–742.

Chaudhari S et al. (2000) Mortality and morbidity in high risk infants during a six year follow-up. *Indian Pediatr.* 37(12):1314–1320.

Chaudhari S et al. (2004) Pune low birth weight study cognitive abilities and educational performance at twelve years. *Indian Pediatr.* 2004;41(2):121–128

Chaudhari S et al. (2005) Biology versus environment in low birth weight children. *Indian Pediatr.* 42(8):763–770.

Chen ST (1989) Comparison between the development of Malaysian and Denver children. *J Singapore Paediatr Soc.* 31:178–185.

Chisholm D et al. (2007) Scale up services for mental disorders: a call for action. *Lancet.* 370(9594):1241–1252.

Chitty LS, Winter RM (1989) Perinatal mortality in different ethnic groups. *Arch Dis Child.* 64:1036–1041.

Chopra M (2001) *Assessment of participants on the Care for Development IMCI training course.* University of the Western Cape, Cape Town, South Africa.

Chopra G, Verma IC, Seetharaman P (1999) Development and assessment of a screening test for detecting childhood disabilities. *Indian J Pediatr.* 66(3):331–335.

Chu MM et al. (2006) Modified symbolic play test for Oriental children. *Pediatr Int.* 48(6):519–524.

Cicchetti D, Rogosch F, Toth SL (1998) Maternal depressive disorder and contextual risk: contributions to the development of attachment insecurity and behavior problems in toddlerhood. *Dev Psychopathol.* 10(2):283–300.

Coley RL, Chase-Lansdale PL (1998) Adolescent pregnancy and parenthood: recent evidence and future directions. *Am Psychol.* 53:152–166.

Colleta ND (1983) At risk for depression: a study of young mothers. *J GenetPsychol.* 142: 301–310.

Committee on Hospital Care, American Academy of Pediatrics (2003) Family-centered care and the pediatrician's role. *Pediatrics.* 112: 691–696.

Committee on Nervous System Disorders in Developing Countries (2001) Board on Global Health. *Neurological, psychiatric, and developmental disorders: meeting the challenge in the developing world.* Washington, DC: National Academy Press, 2001

Conway AM, McDonough SC (2006) Emotional resilience in early childhood: developmental antecedents and relations to behavior problems. *Ann NY Acad Sci.* 1094:272–277.

Cooper PA, Sandler DL (1997) Outcome of very low birth weight infants at 12 to 18 months of age in Soweto, South Africa. *Pediatrics.* 99(4):537–544.

Cooper PJ et al. (2002) Impact of a mother-infant intervention in an indigent peri-urban South African context. *Br J Psychiatry.* 180: 76–81.

Corapci F, Radan AE, Lozoff B (2006) Iron deficiency in infancy and mother-child interaction at 5 years. *J Dev Behav Pediatr.* 27:371–378.

Corry PC (2002) Intellectual disability and cerebral palsy in a UK community. *Community Genet.* 5(3):201–204.

Council on Children With Disabilities (2006) Section on Developmental Behavioral Pediatrics, Bright Futures Steering Committee, and Medical Home Initiatives for Children With Special Needs Project Advisory Committee. Identifying infants and young children with developmental disorders in the medical home: an algorithm for developmental surveillance and screening. *Pediatrics.* 118:405–420.

Crishna B (1999) What is community-based rehabilitation? A view from experience. *Child Care Health Dev.* 25(1):27–35.

Currie ML, Rademacher R (2004) The pediatrician's role in recognizing and intervening in postpartum depression. *Pediatr Clin North Am.* 51(3):785–801, xi.

Custers JW et al. (2002) Discriminative validity of the Dutch Pediatric Evaluation of Disability Inventory. *Arch Phys Med Rehabil.* 83(10): 1437–1441.

Daley TC, Sigman MD (2002) Diagnostic conceptualization of autism among Indian psychiatrists, psychologists, and pediatricians. *J Autism Dev Disord.* 32(1):13–23.

Darmstadt GL et al. (2005) Evidence-based, cost-effective interventions: how many newborn babies can we save? *Lancet.* 365(9463):977–988.

Darr A, Modell B (1988) The frequency of consanguineous marriage among British Pakistanis. *J Med Genet.* 25(3):186–190.

Darwin C (1877) A biographical sketch of an infant. A quarterly review of psychology and philosophy. *Mind.* 2: 285–294.

Davis DW et al. (2005) Visual perceptual skills in children born with very low birth weights. *J Pediatr Health Care.* 6:363–367.

Davis H, Tsiantis J (2005) Promoting children's mental health: the European Early Promotion Project (EEPP). *International Journal of Mental Health Promotion.* 7:4–16.

Dawson G, Ashman SB, Carver LJ (2000) The role of early experience in shaping behavioral and brain development and its implications for social policy. *Dev Psychopathol.* 12(4):695–712.

de Lourdes Drachler M et al. (2005) Social inequalities in maternal opinion of child development in southern Brazil. *Acta Paediatr.* 94(8):1006–1008.

de Onis M, Garza C, Victora CG (2003) The WHO Multicentre Growth Reference Study: strategy for developing a new international growth reference. *Forum Nutr.* 56:238–240.

de Onis M et al. (2006) Comparison of the World Health Organization (WHO) Child Growth Standards and the National Center for Health Statistics/WHO international growth reference: implications for child health programmes. *Public Health Nutr.* 9(7):942–947.

de Onis M et al. (2007) Development of a WHO growth reference for school-aged children and adolescents. *Bull World Health Organ.* 85(9):660–667.

DeSouza N et al. (2000) Determinants of follow-up in an early intervention program in high-risk babies. *Indian Pediatr.* 37(9): 986–989.

DeSouza N et al. (2006) The determinants of compliance with an early intervention programme for high-risk babies in India. *Child Care Health Dev.* 32(1): 63–72.

Dhanda A (2007) Mental health and human rights. *Lancet.* 370(9594):1197–1198.

Dinkevich E, Ozuah PO (2002) Well-child care: effectiveness of current recommendations. *Clin Pediatr (Phila).* 41(4):211–217.

Diop B et al. (1982) Diagnosis and symptoms of mental disorder in a rural area of Senegal. *Afr J Med Sci.* 11(3):95–103.

DiPietro JA (2000) Baby and the brain: advances in child development. *Annu Rev Public Health.* 21:455–471.

Dixit A, Govil S, Patel NV (1992) Culture appropriate indicators for monitoring growth and development of urban and rural children below 6 years. *Indian Pediatr.* 29(3):291–299.

Dolva AS, Coster W, Lilja M (2004) Functional performance in children with Down syndrome. *Am J Occup Ther.* 58(6):621–629.

Dos Santos I et al. (1999) Pilot test of the child development of the IMCI "Counsel the mother" module. Study results and recommendations. Pelotas, Brazil.

Downe SM, Butler E, Hinder S (2007) Screening tools for depressed mood after childbirth in UK-based South Asian women: a systematic review. *J Adv Nurs.* 57(6):565–583.

Drachler M de L, Marshall T, de Carvalho Leite JC (2007) A continuous-scale measure of child development for population-based epidemiological surveys: a preliminary study using Item Response Theory for the Denver Test. *Paediatr Perinat Epidemiol.* 21(2):138–153.

Drotar D et al. (1999) Neurodevelopmental outcomes of Ugandan infants with HIV infection: an application of growth curve analysis. *Health Psychol.* 18(2): 114–121.

Dunst CJ, Storck A, Snyder D (2006) Reliability and validity of the DC: 0–3 diagnostic classification system. Bridges practice-based research syntheses. *Research and Training Center on Early Childhood Development.* 4(6): 1–20.

Durkin MS, Hasan ZM, Hasan KZ (1995) The ten questions screen for childhood disabilities: Its uses and limitations in Pakistan. *J Epidemiol Community Health.* 49:431–436.

Durkin MS et al. (2000) Prenatal and postnatal risk factors for mental retardation among children in Bangladesh. *Am J Epidemiol.* 152(11):1024–1033.

Durkin MS et al. (2006) Learning and developmental disabilities. In: Jamison DT et al., eds. *Disease control priorities in developing countries*, 2nd ed. New York, Oxford University Press: 933–951.

Dworkin PH (1989) British and American recommendations for developmental monitoring: the role of surveillance. *Pediatrics.* 84(6):1000–1010.

Dworkin PH (2004) 2003 C. Anderson Aldrich award lecture: enhancing developmental services in child health supervision – an idea whose time has truly arrived. *Pediatrics.* 114(3):827–831.

Dworkin PH (2006) Promoting development through child health services. Introduction to the Help Me Grow roundtable. *J Dev Behav Pediatr.* 27(1 Suppl):S2-4; discussion S17–21, S50–52.

Eapen V, Zoubeidi T, Yunis F (2004) Screening for language delay in the United Arab Emirates. *Child Care Health Dev.* 30(5):541–549.

Earls MF, Hay SS (2006) Setting the stage for success: implementation of developmental and behavioral screening and surveillance in primary care practice – the North Carolina Assuring Better Child Health and Development (ABCD) Project. *Pediatrics.* 118:e183–188.

Egan DF, Brown R (1984) Developmental assessment: 18 months to 4 ½ years. The Bus Puzzle Test. *Child Care, Health Dev.* 10(3): 163–179.

Eickmann SH et al. (2003) Improved cognitive and motor development in a community-based intervention of psychosocial stimulation in northeast Brazil. *Dev Med Child Neurol.* 45(8):536–541.

Eickmann SH et al. (2007) Breast feeding and mental and motor development at 12 months in a low-income population in northeast Brazil. *Paediatr Perinat Epidemiol.* 21(2):129–137.

Elder MJ, De Cock R (1993) Childhood blindness in the West Bank and Gaza Strip: prevalence, aetiology and hereditary factors. *Eye.* 7:580–583.

Elster AB, McAnarney ER, Lamb ME (1983) Parental behavior of adolescent mothers. *Pediatrics.* 71(4):494–503.

Emde RN, Wise BK (2003) The cup is half full: initial clinical trials of DC: 0–3 and a recommendation for revision. *Infant Ment Health J.* 24(4):437–446.

Engel G (1977). The need for a new medical model: a challenge for biomedicine. *Science.* 196:129–136.

Engle PL (1993) Influences of mothers'and fathers' income on children's nutritional status in Guatemala. *Soc Sci Med.* 37(11):1303–1312.

Engle PL, Smidt RK (1996) *Influences of adolescent childbearing and marital status at first birth on rural Guatemalan women and children*. Report prepared under the Population Council/ICRW joint program, Family structure, female headship and maintenance of families and poverty.New York and Washington, DC: The Population Council and ICRW.

Engle PL, Castle S, Menon P (1996) Child development: vulnerability and resilience. *Soc Sci Med.* 43(5):621–635.

Engle PL et al. (2007) Strategies to avoid the loss of developmental potential in more than 200 million children in the developing world. *Lancet.* 369:229–242.

Erkin G et al. (2007) Validity and reliability of the Turkish translation of the Pediatric Evaluation of Disability Inventory (PEDI). *Disabil Rehabil.* 29(16): 1271–1279.

Ertem IO (2011). Monitoring and Supporting Early Childhood Development. In: *Rudolph's Pediatrics* 22nd Edition. Rudolph CD, Rudolph AM, Lister GE, First l, Gershon AA (Eds). New York: McGraw-Hill 2011:34–38.

Ertem IO et al. (1997) Development of a supplement to the HOME Scale for children living in impoverished urban environments. *J Dev Behav Pediatr.* 18(5):322–328.

Ertem IO et al. (2006) Promoting child development at sick-child visits: a controlled trial. *Pediatrics.*118:e124–131.

Ertem IO et al. (2007) Mothers' knowledge of young child development in a developing country. *Child Care Health Dev.*33 :728 –737.

Ertem IO et al. (2008) A guide for monitoring child development in low- and middle-income countries. *Pediatrics.* 121(3):e581–589.

Ertem IO et al. (2009) Addressing early childhood development in primary health care: experience from a middle-income country. *J Dev Behav Pediatr.* 30(4):319–326.

Eshel N et al. (2006) Responsive parenting: interventions and outcomes. *Bull World Health Organization* 84: 992–999.

European Agency for Development in Special Needs Education (2005) *Early childhood intervention: analysis of situations in Europe.* (http://www.european-agency.org/publications/ereports/early-childhood-intervention/eci_en.pdf).

Figueiras AC et al. (2003) Evaluation of practices and knowledge among primary health care professionals in relation to child development surveillance. *Cad Saude Publica.* 19(6):1691–1699.

Finkenflügel H, Wolffers I, Huijsman R (2005) The evidence base for community-based rehabilitation: a literature review. *Int J Rehabil Res.* 28(3): 187–201.

Finkenflügel HJ et al. (1996) Appreciation of community-based rehabilitation by caregivers of children with a disability. *Disabil Rehabil.* 18(5):255–260.

Fisher RP, McCauley ML (1995) Information retrieval: interviewing witnesses. In: Brewer N, Wilson C, eds. *Psychology and policing.* Hillsdale, NJ: Erlbaum:81–99.

Forsyth BW (2000) The AIDS epidemic. Past and future. *Child Adolesc Psychiatr Clin N Am.* 9(2):267–278.

Forsyth BW (2003) Psychological aspects of HIV infection in children. *Child Adolesc Psychiatr Clin N Am.* 12(3):423–437.

Forsyth BW et al. (1996) The psychological effects of parental human immunodeficiency virus infection on uninfected children. *Arch Pediatr Adolesc Med.* 150(10):1015–1020.

Frankenburg WK et al. (1992) The Denver II: a major revision and restandardization of the Denver Developmental Screening Test. *Pediatrics.* 89:91– 97.

Frankenburg WK, Dodds JB (1967) The Denver developmental screening test. *J Pediatr.* 71(2):181–191.

Freire-Maia N, Elisbao T (1984) Inbreeding effect on morbidity: a review of the world literature. *Am J Med Genet.* 18:391–400.

Friedman SB (1970) The challenge in behavioral pediatrics. *J Pediatr.* 77:172.

Friedman SB, ed. (1975) Introduction: behavioral pediatrics. *Pediatr Clin N Am.* 22:55.

Furstenburg FF, Brooks-Gunn J, Morgan SP (1987) *Adolescent mothers in later life.* New York, Cambridge University Press.

REFERENCES

Gannotti ME, Cruz C (2001) Content and construct validity of a Spanish translation of the Pediatric Evaluation of Disability Inventory for children living in Puerto Rico. *Phys Occup Ther Pediatr.* 20(4): 7–24.

Garcia Coll C, Magnuson K (2000) Cultural differences as sources of developmental vulnerabilities and resources. In: Shonkoff JP, Meisels SJ, eds. *Handbook of early childhood*, 2nd ed. Cambridge, Cambridge University Press: 94–114.

Garg P, Bolisetty S (2007) Neonatology in developed and developing nations. *Indian J Pediatr.* 74(2):169–171.

George R, Lee B (1997). Abuse and neglect of the children. In: Maynard R, ed. *Kids having kids: the economic costs and social consequences of teen pregnancy.* Washington, DC: Urban Institute Press: 205–230.

Gillette Y et al. (1991) Hospital-based case management for medically fragile infants: program design. *Patient Educ Couns.* 17(1): 49–58.

Gilliam WS, Meisels SJ, Mayes LC (2005) Screening and surveillance in early intervention systems. In: Guralnick MJ, ed. *The developmental systems approach to early intervention.* Baltimore, MD: Paul H. Brookes: 73–98.

Gilliam WS et al. (2000) Evaluating child and family demonstration initiatives: lessons from the Comprehensive Child Development Program. *Early Child Res Q.* 15:41–45.

Gladstone M et al. (2008) Can Western developmental screening tools be modified for use in a rural Malawian setting? *Arch Dis Child.* 93(1):23–29.

Glascoe FP (1996) *Technical manual for the Brigance Screening Tests.* North Billerica, Massachusetts, Curriculum Associates Inc.

Glascoe FP (2001) Are overreferrals on developmental screening tests really a problem? *Arch Pediatr Adolesc Med.* 155(1):54–59.

Glascoe FP (2002) *Collaborating with parents: using Parents' Evaluation of Developmental Status (PEDS) to detect and address developmental and behavioral problems.* Nashville, TN: Ellsworth & Vandermeer Press LLC.

Glascoe FP (2005) Screening for developmental and behavioral problems. *Ment Retard Dev Disabil Res Rev.* 11:173–179.

Glascoe FP et al. (1992) Accuracy of the Denver-II in developmental screening. *Pediatrics.* 89(6 pt 2):1221–1225.

Glascoe FP et al. (1998) Brief approaches to educating patients and parents in primary care. *Pediatrics.* 101(6):E10.

Gona JK, Hartley S, Newton CR (2006) Using participatory rural appraisal (PRA) in the identification of children with disabilities in rural Kilifi, Kenya. *Rural Remote Health.* 6(3):553 (Epub 2006 Sep 6).

Gordis L, Markowitz M (1971) Evaluation of the effectiveness of comprehensive and continuous pediatric care. *Pediatrics.* 48(5):766–776.

Gottlieb CA et al. (2009) Child disability screening, nutrition, and early learning in 18 countries with low and middle incomes: data from the third round of UNICEF's Multiple Indicator Cluster Survey (2005–06). *Lancet.* 374(9704):1831–1839.

Gove S (1997) Integrated management of childhood illness by outpatient health workers: technical basis and overview. The WHO Working Group on Guidelines for Integrated Management of the Sick Child. *Bull World Health Organ.* 75(Suppl 1): 7–24.

Grantham-McGregor S, Baker-Henningham H (2005) Review of the evidence linking protein and energy to mental development. *Public Health Nutr.* 8(7A):1191–1201.

Grantham-McGregor S, Schofield W, Harris L (1983) Effect of psychosocial stimulation on mental development of severely malnourished children: an interim report. *Pediatrics.* 72(2):239–243.

Grantham-McGregor SM, Schofield W, Powell C (1987) Development of severely malnourished children who received psychosocial stimulation: six-year follow-up. *Pediatrics.* 79(2): 247–254.

Grantham-McGregor SM et al. (1991) Nutritional supplementation, psychosocial stimulation, and mental development of stunted children: the Jamaican Study. *Lancet.* 338(8758):1–5.

Grantham-McGregor SM et al. (1998) The development of low birth weight term infants and the effects of the environment in northeast Brazil. *J Pediatr.* 132(4): 661–666.

Grantham-McGregor S et al. (2007) Developmental potential in the first 5 years for children in developing countries. *Lancet.* 369(9555): 60–70.

Graves P, Gelband H (2006) Vaccines for preventing malaria (SPf66). Cochrane Database of Systematic Reviews. Issue 2. Art. No.: CD005966 (DOI: 10.1002/14651858.CD005966).

Gray R, Francis E (2007) The implications of US experiences with early childhood interventions for the UK Sure Start Programme. *Child Care Health Dev.* 33(6): 655–663.

Green M (1994) *Bright futures: guidelines for health supervision of infants, children, and adolescents.* Arlington, VA: National Center for Education in Maternal and Child Health.

Greenough A, Milner A, Dimitriou G (2000) Synchronized mechanical ventilation for respiratory support in newborn infants. *Cochrane Database Syst Rev.* 2: CD000456.

Groce NE, Trani JF (2009) Millennium Development Goals and people with disabilities. *Lancet.* 374:1800–1801.

Gupta R, Patel NV (1991) Trial of a screening technique of the developmental assessment of infants and young children (6 weeks–2 years). *Indian Pediatr.* 28(8):859–867.

Guralnick MJ (1997). The effectiveness of early intervention. Paul H. Brookes Publishing Co., Baltimore, MD.

Guralnick MJ (2005a) *The developmental systems approach to early intervention.* Baltimore, MD: PH Brookes Publishing Co.

Guralnick MJ (2005b) Early intervention for children with intellectual disabilities: current knowledge and future prospects. *J Appl Res Intellect Disabil.* 18:313–324.

Guralnick MJ (2006a) Early intervention/program development. *Journal of Policy and Practice in Intellectual Disabilities.* 3(1):1–3.

Guralnick MJ (2006b) The system of early intervention for children with developmental disabilities: Current status and challenges for the future. In: Jacobson JW, Mulick JA, Rojahn J, eds. *Handbook of mental retardation and developmental disabilities.* New York: Plenum: 465–480.

Hack M et al. (1992) The effect of very low birth weight and social risk on neurocognitive abilities at school age. *J Dev Behav Pediatr.* 13(6): 412–420.

Hafez M et al. (1985) Autosomal recessive genes causing mental deficiency in Egyptian children. *Egyptian journal of genetics and cytology.* 14: 259–264.

Hagan JF, Shaw S, Duncan P, eds. (2008) *Bright futures: guidelines for health supervision of infants, children, and adolescents*, 3rd ed. Elk Grove Village, IL: American Academy of Pediatrics.

Haggerty RJ, Friedman SB (2003) History of developmental-behavioral pediatrics. *J Dev Behav Pediatr.* 24:1–18.

Haggman-Laitila A (2003) Early support needs of Finnish families with small children. *J Adv Nurs.* 41(6):595–606.

Haley SM et al. (2004) Pediatric physical functioning reference curves. *Pediatr Neurol.* 31(5):333–341.

Halfon N et al. (2004) Assessing development in the pediatric office. *Pediatrics.* 113(6 Suppl):1926–1933.

Hall DR, Smith M, Smith J (1996) Maternal factors contributing to asphyxia neonatorum. *J Trop Pediatr.* 42:192–195.

Halliday HI, Ehrenkrantz RA (2000) Early postnatal corticosteroids for preventing chronic lung disease in preterm infants. *Cochrane Database Syst Rev.* 2: CD001146.

Hamadani JD et al. (2002) Zinc supplementation during pregnancy and effects on mental development and behaviour of infants: a follow-up study. *Lancet.* 360(9329): 290–294.

Hamadani JD et al. (2006) Psychosocial stimulation improves the development of undernourished children in rural Bangladesh. *J Nutr.* 136(10):2645–2652.

Hannon P (2003) Developmental neuroscience implications for early childhood intervention and education. *Current Paediatrics.* 13: 58–63.

Hariyono R et al. (1987) Denver Developmental Screening Test on children in the Well-Baby Clinic, Dr. Kariadi Hospital Semarang, Indonesia. *Paediatr Indones.* 27(5–6):85–92.

Hartley S et al. (2005) How do carers of disabled children cope? The Ugandan perspective. *Child Care Health Dev.* 31(2):167–180.

Hashemipour M et al. (2007) Parental consanguinity among parents of neonates with congenital hypothyroidism in Isfahan. *East Mediterr Health J.* 13(3):567–574.

Haskett ME, Johnson CA, Miller JW (1994) Individual differences in risk of child abuse by adolescent mothers: assessment in the perinatal period. *J Child Psychol Psychiatry.* 35: 461–476.

Hayes H et al. (2006) Short birth intervals and the risk of school unreadiness among a Medicaid population in South Carolina. *Child Care Health Dev.* 32(4):423–430.

Helander E, Mendis P, Nelson G (1980) *Training disabled people in the community.* Geneva, World Health Organization.

Helander E, Mendis P, Nelson G (1989) *Training disabled people in the community*, revised edition. Geneva, World Health Organization.

Henderson-Smart DJ et al. (2000) Elective high frequency oscillatory ventilation for acute pulmonary dysfunction in preterm infants. *Cochrane Database Syst Rev.* 2: CD000104.

Herrman H, Swartz L (2007) Promotion of mental health in poorly resourced countries. *Lancet.* 370(9594): 1195–1197.

Hertzman C, Power C (2004) Child development as a determinant of health across the life course. *Current Paediatrics.* 14:438–443.

Heymann J (2006) *Forgotten families: ending the growing confrontation children and working parents in the global economy*. New York: Oxford University Press.

Hill JL, Brooks-Gunn J, Waldfogel J (2003) Sustained effects of high participation in an early intervention for low-birth-weight premature infants. *Dev Psychol*. 39(4):730–744.

Hill Z, Kirkwood B, Edmond K (2004) *Family and community practices that promote child survival, growth and development. A review of the evidence*. Geneva, World Health Organization.

Ho JJ et al. (1999) Neurodevelopmental outcome of very low birth weight babies admitted to a Malaysian nursery. *J Paediatr Child Health*. 35(2):175–180.

Hook EB (1982) Incidence and prevalence as measures of the frequency of birth defects. *Am J Epidemiol*. 116:743–747.

Hornby SJ et al. (2000) Requirements for optical services in children with microphthalmos, coloboma and microcornea in southern India. *Eye*. 14(Pt 2):219–224.

Hornstein J, O'Brien MA, Stadtler AC (1997) Touchpoints practice: lessons learned from training and implementation. *Zero to Three*. 17 (6): 26–31.

Horowitz FD et al. (1977) The effects of obstetrical medication on the behavior of Israeli newborn infants and some comparisons with Uruguayan and American infants. *Child Dev*. 48(4):1607–1623.

Horton R (2007) Launching a new movement for mental health. *Lancet*. 370(9590):806.

House H, McAlister M, Naidoo C (1990) *Zimbabwe steps ahead: community rehabilitation and people with disabilities*. London, Catholic Institute for International Relations.

Hubbs-Tait L et al. (1994) Predicting behavior problems and social competence in children of adolescent mothers. *Fam Relat*. 43:439–446.

Hutton G (2006) *The effect of maternal-newborn health on households: economic vulnerability and social implications*. Geneva, World Health Organization (Moving Towards Universal Coverage. Issues in Maternal-Newborn Health and Poverty, No. 1).

Ilett SJ (1995) Putting it on tape: audio taped assessment summaries for parents. *Arch Dis Child*. 73(5):435–438.

Infant Health and Development Program (1990). Enhancing the outcomes of low birth weight, premature infants: a multisite, randomized trial. *J Am Med Assoc*. 263:3035–3042.

IPSCAN (2008) *World perspectives on child abuse. An international resource book*, 8th ed. Chicago: IPSCAN Publications (http://www.ispcan.org/wp/index.htm).

Iranfar S et al. (2005) Is unintended pregnancy a risk factor for depression in Iranian women? *East Mediterr Health J*. 11(4):618–624.

Irwin LG, Siddiqi A, Hertzman C (2007) *Early child development: a powerful equalizer*. Final report for the World Health Organization's Commission on Social Determinants of Health. Geneva, World Health Organization (http://www.who.int/social_determinants/resources/ecd_kn_report_07_2007.pdf).

Ivanans T (1975) Effect of maternal education and ethnic background on infant development. *Arch Dis Child*. 50(6):454–457.

Izuora GI (1985) Aetiology of mental retardation in Nigerian children around Enugu. *Cent Afr J Med*. 31(1):13–16.

Jaber L et al. (1992) Marked parental consanguinity as a cause for increased major malformations in an Israeli Arab community. *Am J Med Genet*. 44:1–6.

Jacob KS et al. (2007) Mental health systems in countries: where are we now? *Lancet*. 370(9592):1061–1077.

Jakob R et al. (2007) The WHO Family of International Classifications. *Bundesgesundheitsblatt Gesundheitsforschung Gesundheitsschutz*. 50(7): 924–931.

Jamison DT et al., eds. (2006) *Disease control priorities in developing countries*, 2nd ed. New York: Oxford University Press: 933–951.

Jaruratanasirikul S et al. (2004) Clinical abnormalities, intervention program, and school attendance of Down syndrome children in southern Thailand. *J Med Assoc Thai*. 87(10):1199–1204.

Jobe AH (1993) Pulmonary surfactant therapy. *N Engl J Med*. 328:861–868.

Jones DJ et al. (2002) Positive parenting and child psychosocial adjustment in inner-city single-parent African American families. The role of maternal optimism. *Behav Modif*. 26(4):464–481.

Jongmans M et al. (1997) Minor neurological signs and perceptual-motor difficulties in prematurely born children. *Arch Dis Child*. 76:9–14.

Joyce TJ, Kaestner R, Korenman S (2000) The effect of pregnancy intention on child development. *Demography*. 37(1):83–94.

Kabarity A et al. (1981) Autosomal recessive "uncomplicated" profound childhood deafness in an Arabic family with high consanguinity. *Hum Genet*. 57:444–446.

Kabiri M (1982) A report on the incidence of phenylketonuria (PKU) in Teheran, Iran. *Acta Med Iran*. 24:127–113.

Kalra V, Seth R, Sapra S (2005) Autism-experiences in a tertiary care hospital. *Indian J Pediatr*. 72:227–230.

Karamizadeh Z, Amrihakimi G (1992) Incidence of congenital hypothyroidism in Fars Province, Iran. *Iranian journal of medical sciences*. 17(1&2):78–80.

Katonka S (2007) Users' networks for Africans with mental disorders. *Lancet*. 370(9591): 919–920.

Katz M et al. (2002) Demography of pediatric primary care in Europe: delivery of care and training. *Pediatrics*. 109(5):788–796.

Kaul S et al. (2003) Working with families to implement home interventions: India. In: Odom SL et al. eds. *Early intervention practices around the world*. Baltimore, MD: Paul H. Brookes: 111–129.

Keefer CH et al. (1982) Specific differences in motor performance between Gusii and American newborns and a modification of the Neonatal Behavioral Assessment Scale. *Child Dev*. 53(3):754–759.

Kelly A (2007) *Evidence review: Prevention of disabilities*. Population Health and Wellness. Core Public Health Functions for BC, Ministry of Health, Vancouver, British Columbia, Canada.

Kerber KJ et al. (2007) Continuum of care for maternal, newborn, and child health: from slogan to service delivery. *Lancet*. 370(9595):1358–1369.

Khan D (2004) Adolescent pregnancy: unmet needs and undone deeds. A review of the literature and programmes. Geneva, World Health Organization.

Khan MA (1992) Intellectual and developmental assessment of cerebral palsy cases in Libyan City. *Indian J Med Sci*. 46(8):235–238.

Khan NZ et al. (1998) Mortality of urban and rural young children with cerebral palsy in Bangladesh. *Dev Med Child Neurol*. 40(11): 749–753.

Khan NZ et al. (2006) Neurodevelopmental outcomes of preterm infants in Bangladesh. *Pediatrics*. 118: 280–289.

Khouzam N, Chenouda E, Naguib G (2003) A family partnership model of early intervention: Egypt. In: Odom SL et al., eds. *Early intervention practices around the world*. Baltimore: Paul H. Brookes: 151–171.

Khrouf N et al. (1986) Malformations in 10 000 consecutive births in Tunis. *Acta Paediatr Scand*. 75:534–539.

Kinoti SN (1993) Asphyxia of the newborn in east, central and southern Africa. *East Afr Med J*. 70(7): 422–433.

Kirksey A et al. (1994) Relation of maternal zinc nutriture to pregnancy outcome and infant development in an Egyptian village. *Am J Clin Nutr*. 60(5):782–792.

Kirsten GF et al. (1995) The outcome at 12 months of very low birth weight infants ventilated at Tygeberg Hospital. *S Afr Med J*. 85(7):649–654.

Klebanov P, Brooks-Gunn J (2006) Cumulative, human capital, and psychological risk in the context of early intervention: links with IQ at ages 3, 5, and 8. *Ann N Y Acad Sci*. 1094:63–82.

Klinnert MD et al. (2001) Onset and persistence of childhood asthma: predictors from infancy. *Pediatrics*. 108(4):E69.

Knight J, Frazer C, Emans SJ (2001). Bright Futures case studies for primary care clinicians: child development and behavior. Boston, MA: Bright Futures Center for Education in Child Growth and Development, Behavior and Adolescent Health.

Knight JR et al. (2001) Development of a Bright Futures curriculum for pediatric residents. *Ambul Pediatr*. 1(3):136–140.

Knippenberg R et al. (2005) Systematic scaling up of neonatal care in countries. *Lancet*. 365(9464):1087–1098.

Korenman S, Kaestner R, Joyce T (2002) Consequences for infants of parental disagreement in pregnancy intention. *Perspect Sex Reprod Health*. 34(4):198–205.

Kraemer HC, Fendt KH (1990) Random assignment in clinical trials: issues in planning (Infant Health and Development Program). *J Clin Epidemiol*. 43(11):1157–1167.

Krishnaswamy J (1992) The UPANAYAN early intervention programme. *Indian J Pediatr*. 59(6):701–705.

Krishnaswamy MJ (1994) *Computer assisted training programme for early intervention for children with mental retardation*. Berlin/Heidelberg, Springer: 616–620.

Kukuruza A (1998) *The concept of an early intervention center for children with disability and developmental delays*. Central European University Center For Policy Studies (http://pdc.ceu.hu/archive/00001925/01/kukuruza.pdf ; accessed 20 June 2008)

Kuliev AM (1986) Thalassaemia can be prevented. *World Health Forum*. 7:286–290.

Kumar R et al. (1997) Factors influencing psychosocial development of preschool children in a rural area of Haryana, India. *J Trop Pediatr*. 43(6):324–329.

Kuo AA et al. (2006) Rethinking well-child care in the United States: an international comparison. *Pediatrics*. 118(4):1692–1702.

Kuruvilla S, Joseph A (1999) Identifying disability: comparing house-to-house survey and rapid rural appraisal. *Health Policy and Planning*. 14, 182–190.

Lambrechts T, Bryce J, Orinda V (1999) Integrated management of childhood illness: a summary of first experiences. *Bull World Health Organ*. 77(7):582–594.

REFERENCES

Lansdown RG, Goldstein H, Shah PM, Orley JH, Di G, Kaul KK, Kumar V, Laksanavicharn U, Reddy V (1996) Culturally appropriate measures for monitoring child development at family and community level: a WHO collaborative study. *Bull World Health Organ.* 74(3):283–90.

Lau KM, Chow SM, Lo SK (2006) Parents' perceptions of the quality of life of preschool children at risk or having developmental disabilities. *Qual of Life Res.* 15(7): 1133–1141.

Lavi E, Rosenberg J (2005) Disclosure of severe development disability: a survey of parents' experiences and preferences at an Israeli child development center. *Harefuah.* 144(5):453–458.

Lawn J, Shibuya K, Stein C (2005) No cry at birth global estimates of intrapartum stillbirths and intrapartum-related neonatal deaths. *Bull World Health Organ.* 83:409–417.

Lawn JE et al. (2005) 4 million neonatal deaths: When? Where? Why? *Lancet.* 365(9462):891–900.

Lawrie TA et al. (1998) Validation of the Edinburgh Postnatal Depression Scale on a cohort of South African women. *S Afr Med J.* 88(10): 1340–1344.

Leadbeater BJ, Bishop SJ, Raver CC (1996) Quality of mother-child interactions, maternal depressive symptoms and behavior problems in preschoolers of adolescent mothers. *Dev Psychol.* 32:280–288.

Lee DT et al. (1998) Detecting postnatal depression in Chinese women. Validation of the Chinese version of the Edinburgh Postnatal Depression Scale. *Br J Psychiatry.* 172: 433–437.

Lejarraga H et al. (2002) Psychomotor development in Argentinean children aged 0–5 years. *Paediatr Perinat Epidemiol.* 16:47–60.

Lester BM, Masten A, McEwen B, eds. (2006) Resilience in children. *Annals of the New York Academy of Sciences*, December 2006, Vol. 1094.

Lequerica M (1997) Toward a one-stop model of service for low- income preschoolers: insights from clinical practice and research. *Infant-Toddler Intervention.* 7(4); 295–300.

Li Y et al. (2000) Maternal child rearing behaviors and correlates in rural minority areas of Yunnan, China. *J Dev Behav Pediatr.* 21:114–122.

Lian WB et al. (2003) General practitioners' knowledge on childhood developmental and behavioural disorders. *Singapore Med J.* 44(8):397–403.

Liao HF, Pan YL (2005) Test–retest and inter-rater reliability for the Comprehensive Developmental Inventory for Infants and Toddlers diagnostic and screening tests. *Early Hum Dev.* 81(11):927–937.

Liao HF et al. (2005) Concurrent validity of the Comprehensive Developmental Inventory for Infants and Toddlers with the Bayley Scales of Infant Development-II in preterm infants. *J Formos Med Assoc.* 104(10):731–737.

Lim HC, Chan T, Yoong T (1994) Standardisation and adaptation of the Denver Developmental Screening Test (DDST) and Denver II for use in Singapore children. *Singapore Med J.* 35(2):156–160.

Lima MC et al. (2004) Determinants of mental and motor development at 12 months in a low income population: a cohort study in northeast Brazil. *Acta Paediatr.* 93(7):969–975.

Lloyd CB, ed. (2005) Growing up global: the challenging transitions to adulthood in developing countries. Panel on Transitions to Adulthood in Developing Countries. Committee on Population. Board on Children, Youth, and Families. Division of Behavioral and Social Sciences and Education. *National Research Council and Institute of Medicine of The National Academies. Washington, DC, National Academies Press.*

Logan 1995 Early Identification of impairments in children (pg 101–110). In *Disabled Children in Developing Countries.* Pam Zinkin, Helen McConachie (Eds), Mac Keith Press, London.

Lollar DJ, Simeonsson RJ (2005) Diagnosis to function: classification for children and youths. *J Dev Behav Pediatr.* 26(4): 323–330.

López Stewart C et al. (2000) Parenting and physical punishment: primary care interventions in Latin America. *Rev Panam Salud Publica.* 8(4):257–267.

Louw B, Avenant C (2002) Culture as context for intervention: developing a culturally congruent early intervention program. *Int Pediatr.* 17(3):145–150.

Love JM et al. (2005) The effectiveness of early head start for 3-year-old children and their parents: lessons for policy and programs. *Dev Psychol.* 41(6):885–901.

Lowe M, Costello A (1976) *Manual for symbolic play test.* London: National Foundation of Educational Research.

Lozoff B, Georgieff MK (2006) Iron deficiency and brain development. *Semin Pediatr Neurol.* 13(3):158–165.

Lozoff B, Jimenez E, Smith JB (2006) Double burden of iron deficiency in infancy and low socioeconomic status: a longitudinal analysis of cognitive test scores to age 19 years. *Arch Pediatr Adolesc Med.* 160(11):1108–1113.

Lubbe W (2005) Early intervention care programme for parents of neonates. *Curationis.* 28(3):54–63.

Lumpkin GH, Aranha MSF (2003) The right to a good and supportive start in life: Brazil. In: Odom SL et al., eds. *Early intervention practices around the world.* Baltimore: Paul H. Brookes: 129–151.

Lyons-Ruth K, Block D (1996) The disturbed caregiving systems: Relations among childhood trauma, maternal caregiving, and infant affect and attachment. *Infant Ment Health J.* 17: 257–275.

Magill-Evans J, Hodge M, Darrah J (2002) Establishing a transdisciplinary research team in academia. *J Allied Health.* 31:222–226.

Malhi P, Singhi P (2002) Role of parents' evaluation of developmental status in detecting developmental delay in young children. *Indian Pediatr.* 39(3):271–275.

Margolis PA et al. (2001) From concept to application: the impact of a community-wide intervention to improve the delivery of preventive services to children. *Pediatrics.* 108(3):E42.

Marlow N (2004) Neurocognitive outcome after very preterm birth. *Arch Dis Child Fetal Neonatal Ed.* 89(3): F224–228.

Martines J et al. (2005) Neonatal survival: a call for action. *Lancet.* 365(9465):1189–1197.

Mathur GP et al. (1995) Detection and prevention of childhood disability with the help of Anganwadi workers. *Indian Pediatr.* 32 (7):773–777.

Maulik PK, Darmstadt GL (2007) Childhood disability in low- and middle-income countries: overview of screening, prevention, services, legislation, and epidemiology. *Pediatrics.* 120 Suppl 1:S1–55.

Mayor S (2004) Pregnancy and childbirth are leading causes of death in teenage girls in developing countries. *BMJ.* 328(7449):1152.

Mbise AS, Kysela GM (1990) Developing appropriate screening and assessment instruments: the case of Tanzania. In: Thornburn MJ, Marfo K, eds. *Practical approaches to childhood disability in developing countries: Insights from experience and research.* St Johns, Newfoundland: Memorial University, Project SEDEREC, Spanish Town Jamaica: 3D Projects: 225–243.

McAllister CL et al. (2005) "Come and take a walk": listening to Early Head Start parents on school-readiness as a matter of child, family, and community health. *Am J Public Health.* 95(4): 617–625.

McConachie H et al. (2000) A randomized controlled trial of alternative modes of service provision to young children with cerebral palsy in Bangladesh. *J Pediatr.* 137(6):769–776.

McConachie H et al. (2001) Difficulties for mothers in using an early intervention service for children with cerebral palsy in Bangladesh. *Child Care Health Dev.* 27(1):1–12.

McConkey R (1995) Early intervention in developing countries. In: Zinkin P, McConachie H, eds. *Disabled children and developing countries*, London: MacKeith Press (Clinics in Developmental Medicine No. 136).

McCormick MC et al. (1991) Health care use among young children in day care. Results in a randomized trial of early intervention. *JAMA.* 265(17):2212–2217.

McGrath N et al. (2006) Effect of maternal multivitamin supplementation on the mental and psychomotor development of children who are born to HIV-1-infected mothers in Tanzania. *Pediatrics.* 117(2): e216–225.

McHenry PC et al. (1990) Mediators of depression among low-income, adolescent mothers of infants: a longitudinal perspective. *J Youth Adolesc.* 19: 327–347.

McIntyre P (2006) *Pregnant adolescents: delivering on global promises of hope.* Geneva, World Health Organization.

McKay K (2006) Evaluating model programs to support dissemination. An evaluation of strengthening the developmental surveillance and referral practices of child health providers. *J Dev Behav Pediatr.* 27:S26–S29.

McLearn KT et al. (1998) Child development and pediatrics for the 21st century: the healthy steps approach. *J Urban Health.* 75(4): 704–723.

McLearn KT et al. (2004) Developmental services in primary care for low-income children: clinicians' perceptions of the Healthy Steps for Young Children program. *J Urban Health.* 81:206–221.

Meisels SJ, Atkins-Burnett S (2000) The elements of early childhood assessment. In: Shonkoff JP, Meisels SJ, eds. *Handbook of early childhood intervention.* New York, Cambridge University Press: 231–257.

Meisels SJ, Fenichel ES, eds. (1996) *New visions for the developmental assessment of infants and young children.* Washington, DC: Zero to Three/National Center for Infants, Toddlers, and Families Publications.

Melnyk BM et al. (2004) Creating opportunities for parent empowerment: program effects on the mental health/coping outcomes of critically ill young children and their mothers. *Pediatrics.* 113(6):e597–607.

Milaat WA et al. (2001) Population-based survey of childhood disability in eastern Jeddah using the ten questions tool. *Disabil Rehabil.* 23(5):199–203.

Miller B, Moore K (1990) Adolescent sexual behavior, pregnancy and parenting: research through the 1980s. *J Marriage Fam.* 52:1025–1044.

Miller G (2007) Mental health and the mass media: room for improvement. *Lancet.* 370(9592):1015–1016.

Minde KK (1977) Children in Uganda: rates of behavioural deviations and psychiatric disorders in various school and clinic populations. *J Child Psychol Psychiatry.* 18(1):23–37.

Ministry of Women and Child Development (2009). *Three decades of ICDS – an appraisal.* New Delhi, Government of India (http://wcd.nic.in/3dicds.htm; accsessed 21 June 2009).

Minkovitz C et al. (2001) Early effects of the healthy steps for young children program. *Arc Pediatr Adolesc Med.* 155(4):470–479.

Mobarak R et al. (2000) Predictors of stress in mothers of children with cerebral palsy in Bangladesh. *J Pediatr Psychol.* 25(6): 427–433.

Mohllajee AP et al. (2007) Pregnancy intention and its relationship to birth and maternal outcomes. *Obstet Gynecol.* 109(3):678–686.

Montazeri A, Torkan B, Omidvari S (2007) The Edinburgh Postnatal Depression Scale (EPDS): translation and validation study of the Iranian version. *BMC Psychiatry.* 7:11.

Morton R et al. (2002) Disability in children from different ethnic populations. *Child Care Health Dev.* 28(1):87–93.

Moszynski P (2004) Girls in southern Sudan are more likely to die in childbirth than complete primary school. *BMJ.* 328(7455):1514.

Msall ME (2005) Measuring functional skills in preschool children at risk for neurodevelopmental disabilities. *Ment Retard and Dev Disabil Res Rev.* 11 (3): 263–273.

Msall ME (2006) Neurodevelopmental surveillance in the first 2 years after extremely preterm birth: evidence, challenges, and guidelines. *Early Hum Dev.* 82(3): 157–166.

Msall ME, Tremont MR (2002) Measuring functional outcomes after prematurity: Developmental impact of very low birth weight and extremely low birth weight status on childhood disability. *Ment Retard Dev Disabil Res Rev.* 8:258–272.

Msall ME et al. (1994) The Functional Independence Measure for Children (WeeFIM). Conceptual basis and pilot use in children with developmental disabilities. *Clin Pediatr (Phila).* 33(7):421–430 .

Muhit MA et al. The key informant method: a novel means of ascertaining blind children in Bangladesh. *Br J Ophthalmol.* 91:995–999 (Epub 2007 Apr 12).

Mung'ala-Odera V, Newton CR (2007) Identifying children with neurological impairment and disability in resource-poor countries. *Child Care Health Dev.* 33:249–256. Original Text

Mung'ala-Odera V et al. (2004) Validity and reliability of the 'Ten Questions' questionnaire for detecting moderate to severe neurological impairment in children aged 6–9 years in rural Kenya. *Neuroepidemiology.* 23:67–72.

Murray C, Lopez AD (1994) Quantifying disability: data, methods and results. *Bull World Health Organ.* 71:481–494.

Myers R (1995) *The twelve who survive: strengthening programs of early childhood development in the Third World,* 2nd ed. Ypsilanti, MI: High/Scope Press.

Nair MK et al. (2009) Developmental delay and disability among under-5 children in a rural ICDS block. *Indian Pediatr.* 46 Suppl:75–78.

Nair MK et al. (1991) Trivandrum Developmental Screening Chart. *Indian Pediatr.* 28(8):869–872.

Nasir JA et al. (2004) Investigation of the probable causes of specific childhood disabilities in eastern Afghanistan (preliminary report). *Cent Eur J Public Health.* 12(1):53–57.

Natale JE et al. (1992) Prevalence of childhood disability in a southern Indian city: independent effect of small differences in social status. *Int J Epidemiol.* 21(2):367–372.

National Institute of Health (1995) Consensus Developmental Panel on the Effect of Corticosteroids for Fetal Maturation on Perinatal Outcomes. *JAMA.* 273:413–418.

National Scientific Council on the Developing Child (2007) *The science of early childhood development.* (http://www.developingchild.net; accessed 20 June 2008).

Needleman R et al. (1991) Clinic based intervention to promote literacy. *Am J Dis Child.* 145(8):881–884.

Nelson CA 3rd et al. (2007) Cognitive recovery in socially deprived young children: the Bucharest Early Intervention Project. *Science.* 318(5858):1937–1940.

Neumann C et al. (1991) Relationships between morbidity and development in mildly to moderately malnourished Kenyan toddlers. *Pediatrics.* 88(5): 934–942.

Ngai FW, Wai-Chi Chan S, Holroyd E (2007) Translation and validation of a Chinese version of the parenting sense of competence scale in Chinese mothers. *Nurs Res.* 56(5):348–354.

Niederman LG et al. (2007) Healthy Steps for Young Children program in pediatric residency training: impact on primary care outcomes. *Pediatrics*. 120: e596–e603.

Nyamtema AS, Urassa DP, Roosmalen JV (2011). Maternal health interventions in resource limited countries: a systematic review of packages, impacts and factors for change. *BMC Pregnancy Childbirth*. 17;11(1):30.

O'Brien F et al. (2004) The neurodevelopmental progress of infants less than 33 weeks into adolescence. *Arch Dis Child*. 89 (3):207–211.

O'Connor TG et al. (2000) The effects of global severe privation on cognitive competence: extension and longitudinal follow-up. English and Romanian Adoptees Study Team. *Child Dev*. 71(2):376–390.

Odman P, Krevers B, Oberg B (2007) Parents' perceptions of the quality of two intensive training programmes for children with cerebral palsy. *Dev Med Child Neurol*. 49(2):93–100.

Odom SL et al., eds (2003) *Early intervention practices around the world*. Baltimore: Paul H. Brookes.

Okasha A, Seif el Dawla A (1992) Reliability of ICD-10 research criteria: an Arab perspective. *Acta Psychiatr Scand*. 86(6):484–488.

Olds D (2007) Programs for parents of infants and toddlers: Recent evidence from randomized trials. *J Child Psychol Psychiatry*. 48(3–4):355–391.

Olds DL et al. (2007) Effects of nurse home visiting on maternal and child functioning: age–9 follow-up of a randomized trial. *Pediatrics*. 120(4):e832–845.

Olusanya BO (2007) Promoting effective interventions for neglected health conditions in developing countries. *Disabil Rehabil*. 29(11–12):973–976.

Olusanya BO, Newton VE (2007) Global burden of childhood hearing impairment and disease control priorities for developing countries. *Lancet*. 369(9569):1314–1317.

Omigbodun O et al. (1996) Psychiatric morbidity in a Nigerian paediatric primary care service: a comparison of two screening instruments. *Soc Psychiatry Psychiatr Epidemiol*. 31(3–4):186–193.

Ong LC, Chandran V, Boo NY (2001) Comparison of parenting stress between Malaysian mothers of four-year-old very low birthweight and normal birthweight children. *Acta Paediatr*. 90(12): 1464–1469.

Ong L, Chandran V, Peng R (1999) Stress experienced by mothers of Malaysian children with mental retardation. *J Paediatr Child Health*. 35(4): 358–362.

Ong LC et al. (1998) Parenting stress among mothers of Malaysian children with cerebral palsy: predictors of child-and parent-related stress. *Ann Trop Paediatr*. 18(4): 301–307.

Ostensjo S et al. (2006) Assessment of everyday functioning in young children with disabilities: an ICF-based analysis of concepts and content of the Pediatric Evaluation of Disability Inventory (PEDI). *Disabil Rehabil*. 30,28(8):489–504.

O'Toole B (1989) Community-based rehabilitation for disabled children in rural Guyana. *World Health Forum*. 10(2): 238–239.

O'Toole B, McConkey R (1998) A training strategy for personnel working in developing countries. *Int J Rehabil Res*. 21(3): 311–321.

Ozand T, Devol EB, Generoso GG (1992) Neurometabolic diseases at a national referral centre: five years experience in the King Faisal Specialist Hospital and Research Centre. *J Child Neurol*. 7: Supplement S4–S9.

Özbek A et al. (2005) Development and behavior of non-handicapped preterm children from a developing country. *Pediat Int*. 47 (5):532–540.

Ozguc M et al. (1993) Mutation analysis in Turkish phenylketonuria patients. *J Med Genet*. 30(2):129–131.

Ozmen M et al. (2005) Etiologic evaluation in 247 children with global developmental delay at Istanbul, Turkey. *J Trop Pediatr*. 51(5):310–313 (Epub 2005 Jun 20).

Pal DK et al. (2002) Social integration of children with epilepsy in rural India. *Soc Sci Med*. 54(12):1867–1874.

Palti H, Bendel J, Ornoy A (1992) Prevalence of disabilities in a national sample of 7-year-old Israeli children. *Isr J Med Sci*. 28(7):435–441.

Parker S, Greer S, Zuckerman B (1988) Double jeopardy: the impact of poverty on early child development. *Pediatr Clin North Am*. 35(6):1227–1240.

Patel V (2007) Mental health in low- and middle-income countries. *Br Med Bull*. 81–82:81–96.

Patel V, DeSouza N, Rodrigues M (2003) Postnatal depression and infant growth and development in low income countries: a cohort study from Goa, India. *Arch Dis Child*. 88(1):34–37.

Patel V, Prince M (2006) Maternal psychological morbidity and low birth weight in India. *Br J Psychiatry*. 188:284–285.

Patel V et al. (2007) Treatment and prevention of mental disorders in low-income and middle-income countries. *Lancet*. 370(9591):991–1005.

REFERENCES

Pelto GH et al. (2004) Nutrition counseling training changes physician behavior and improves caregiver knowledge acquisition. *J Nutr.* 134(2):357–362.

Peña ED (2007) Lost in translation: methodological considerations in cross-cultural research. *Child Dev.* 78(4):1255–1264.

Penny N et al. (2007) Community-based rehabilitation and orthopaedic surgery for children with motor impairment in an African context. *Disabil Rehabil.* 29(11–12):839–843.

Phatak AT, Khurana B (1991) Baroda development screening test for infants. *Indian Pediatr.* 28(1):31–37.

Phatak P et al. (1991) A study of Baroda Development Screening Test for infants. *Indian Pediatr.* 28(8):843–849.

Pierson D (1974) The Brooklyn Early Education Project: model for a new education priority. *Childhood Education.* 50:132–136.

Platt MJ et al. (2007). Trends in cerebral palsy among infants of very low birthweight (<1500 g) or born prematurely (<32 weeks) in 16 European centres: a database study. *Lancet.* 369(9555):43–50.

Powell CA et al. (1995) Relationships between physical growth, mental development and nutritional supplementation in stunted children: the Jamaican study. *Acta Paediatr.* 84(1):22–29.

Powell C et al. (2004) Feasibility of integrating early stimulation into primary care for undernourished Jamaican children: cluster randomised controlled trial. *BMJ.* 329(7457):89.

Prathanee B, Dechongkit S, Manochiopinig S (2006) Development of community-based speech therapy model: for children with cleft lip/palate in northeast Thailand. *J Med Assoc Thai.* 89(4): 500–508.

Prince M et al. (2007) No health without mental health. *Lancet.* 370(9590):859–877.

Puura K et al. (2002) The European Early Intervention Promotion Project: A new primary health care service to promote children's mental health. *Infant Mental Health Journal.* 23(6):606–624.

Quiram PA, Capone A Jr (2007) Current understanding and management of retinopathy of prematurity. *Curr Opin Ophthalmol.* 18(3):228–234.

Rahman A et al. (2004a) Impact of maternal depression on infant nutritional status and illness: a cohort study. *Arch Gen Psychiatry.* 61(9): 946–952.

Rahman A et al. (2004b) Mothers' mental health and infant growth: a case-control study from Rawalpindi, Pakistan. *Child Care Health Dev.* 30(1):21–27.

Rahman F et al. (2004c) The magnitude of child injuries in Bangladesh: a major child health problem. *Inj Control Saf Promot.* 11(3):153–157.

Rahman A et al. (2007) Maternal depression increases infant risk of diarrhoeal illness: a cohort study. *Arch Dis Child.* 92(1): 24–28.

Rahman A et al. (2008) Cognitive behaviour therapy-based intervention by community health workers for mothers with depression and their infants in rural Pakistan: a cluster-randomised controlled trial. *Lancet.* 372(9642):902–909.

Raina P et al. (2005) The health and well-being of caregivers of children with cerebral palsy. *Pediatrics.* 115(6): e626–636.

Rajaram P (1990) Child survival: maternal factors. *Indian J Matern Child Health.* 1(2): 39–45.

Ramey CT, Ramey SL (1998) Prevention of intellectual disabilities: early interventions to improve cognitive development. *Prev Med.* 27(2): 224–232.

Ramey CT et al. (1992) Infant Health and Development Program for low birth weight, premature infants: program elements, family participation, and child intelligence. *Pediatrics.* 89(3):454–465.

Regalado M, Halfon N (2001) Primary care services promoting optimal child development from birth to age 3 years: review of the literature. *Arch Pediatr Adolesc Med.* 155:1311–1322.

Reijneveld SA et al. (2004) Identification and management of psychosocial problems among toddlers in Dutch preventive child healthcare. *Arch Pediatr Adolesc Med.* 158:811–817.

Reyes Frausto S et al. (1998) Effect of maternal death on family dynamics and infant survival. *Ginecol Obstet Mex.* 66: 428–433.

Reynell J (1979) *Manual for the Reynell-Zinkin Scales.* London: National Foundation of Education Research.

Richmond JB (1967) Child development: a basic science for pediatrics. *Pediatrics* 39: 649–658.

Richter LM (2003) Occasional article: poverty, underdevelopment and infant mental health. *J Paediatr Child Health.* 39(4): 243–248.

Richter LM (2004) *The importance of caregiver-child interactions for the survival and healthy development of young children: a review.* Geneva: World Health Organization.

Rico JA, Atkin L (1995) *De abuela a madre, de madre a hijos: Repetición intergeneracional del embarazo adolescente y la pobreza.* Report prepared under the Population Council/ICRW joint program, "Family Structure, Female Headship and Maintenance of Families and Poverty." New York and Washington, DC: The Population Council and ICRW.

Roberts H, Hall DMB (2000) What is Sure Start? *Arch Dis Child.* 82: 435–437.

Roberts R et al. (2002) European Early Promotion Project: Transition to Parenting. *Community Pract.* 75:464–468.

Roosa M, Fitzgerald HE, Carlson NA (1982) Teenage parenting and child development: a literature review. *Infant Ment Health J.* 3(1):4–18.

Russell-Brown P, Engle P, Townsend J (1992) *The effects of early childbearing on women's status in Barbados.* Report prepared under the Population Council/ICRW joint program, "Family Structure, Female Headship and Maintenance of Families and Poverty." New York and Washington, DC: The Population Council and ICRW.

Rutstein S (2005) Effects of preceding birth intervals on neonatal, infant and under-five years mortality and nutritional status in developing countries: evidence from the demographic and health surveys. *International Journal of Gynecology & Obstetrics.* 89: S7–S24.

Rutter M (2006) Implications of resilience concepts for scientific understanding. *Ann NY Acad Sci.* 1094:1–12.

Rydz D et al. (2005) Developmental screening. *J Child Neurol.* 20(1):4–21.

Rye H, Hundeide K (2005) Early intervention and children with special needs in developing countries. In: Guralnick MJ, Paul H, eds. *The developmental systems approach to early intervention.* Baltimore, Brookes Publishing Co.: 593–621.

Saeed K et al. (1999) Detection of disabilities by school children: a pilot study in rural Pakistan. *Trop Doct.* 29(3):151–155.

Sameroff AJ, Rosenblum KL (2006) Psychosocial constraints on the development of resilience. *Ann NY Acad Sci.* 1094:116–124.

Sand N et al. (2005) Pediatricians' reported practices regarding developmental screening: do guidelines work? Do they help? *Pediatrics.* 116 (6):174–179.

Saraceno B et al. (2007) Barriers to improvement of mental health services in low-income and middle-income countries. *Lancet.* 370(9593):1164–1174.

Sartorius N (2007) Stigma and mental health. *Lancet.* 370(9590): 810–811.

Sauvey S et al. (2005) Prevalence of childhood and adolescent disabilities in rural Nepal. *Indian Pediatr.* 42(7):697–702.

Save the Children (2001) *Saving newborn lives. The state of the world's newborn: a report from saving newborn lives.* Washington, DC: 1–44.

Saxena S et al. (2007) Resources for mental health: scarcity, inequity, and inefficiency. *Lancet.* 370(9590):878–889.

Schneider E et al. (1995) Performance of Israeli versus U.S. preschool children on the Miller Assessment for Preschoolers. *Am J Occup Ther.* 49:19–23.

Schor EL, Elfenbein C (2004) A need for faculty development in developmental and behavioral pediatrics. *Issue Brief (Commonw Fund).* (785):1–8.

Seligman M, Benjamin Darling R (1989) *Ordinary families, special children: a systems approach to childhood disability.* New York: Guilford Press.

Shah PM et al. (1993) Evaluation of the home-based maternal record: a WHO collaborative study. *Bull World Health Organ.* 71(5):535–48.

Shapira Y, Harel S (1983) Standardization of the Denver developmental screening test for Israeli children. *Isr J Med Sci.* 19(3):246–251.

Shapiro-Mendoza C et al. (2005) Parental pregnancy intention and early childhood stunting: findings from Bolivia. *Int J Epidemiol.* 34(2):387–396.

Sharma, AK et al. (2003) Pregnancy in adolesecnts: a community based study. *Indian Journal of Preventive Social Medicine.* 34 (1&2): 24–32.

Shawky S, Abalkhail B, Soliman N (2002) An epidemiological study of childhood disability in Jeddah, Saudi Arabia. *Paediatr Perinat Epidemiol.* 16(1):61–66.

Shek DT, Lee BM (2007) A comprehensive review of quality of life (QOL) research in Hong Kong. *ScientificWorld Journal.* 17;7:1222–1229.

Shonkoff JP (1993) Reflections on an emerging academic discipline: the prolonged gestation of developmental and behavioral pediatrics. *J Dev Behav Pediatr.* 14(6):409–412.

Shonkoff JP (2006) A promising opportunity for developmental and behavioral pediatrics at the interface of neuroscience, psychology, and social policy: remarks on receiving the 2005 C. Anderson Aldrich Award. *Pediatrics.* 118(5):2187–2191.

Shonkoff JP, Hauser-Cram P (1987) Early intervention for disabled infants and their families: a quantitative analysis. *Pediatrics.* 80:650–658.

Shonkoff JP, Kennell JH (1992) Research in behavioral-developmental pediatrics: new frontiers and elusive boundaries. *Pediatrics.* 90(5 Pt 2):787–788.

Shonkoff JP, Meisels SJ (1990) Preface. In: Meisels SJ, Shonkoff JP, eds. *Handbook of early childhood intervention.* Cambridge, Cambridge University Press.

Shonkoff J, Meisels S, eds. (2000) *Handbook of early childhood intervention*, 2nd ed. New York: Cambridge University Press.

Shonkoff JP, Phillips DA, eds (2000) *From neurons to neighborhoods: the science of early childhood development.* Committee on Integrating the Science of

Early Childhood Development, Board on Children, Youth, and Families. Washington, DC: National Academy Press.

Shonkoff JP, Phillips DA (2001) From neurons to neighborhoods: the science of early childhood development – an introduction. *Zero to Three*. 21(5): 4–7.

Shonkoff JP, Boyce WT, McEwen BS (2009) Neuroscience, molecular biology, and the childhood roots of health disparities: building a new framework for health promotion and disease prevention. *JAMA*. 301(21):2252–2259.

Shore R (1997) *Rethinking the brain: new insights into early development*. New York: Families and Work Institute.

Sices L et al. (2004) How do primary care physicians manage children with possible developmental delays? A national survey with an experimental design. *Pediatrics*. 113:274–282.

Siegel CD et al. (1996) Mortality from intentional and unintentional injury among infants of young mothers in Colorado, 1986 to 1992. *Arch Pediatr Adolesc Med*. 150:1077–1083.

Simeonsson RJ, Scarborough AA, Hebbeler KM (2006) ICF and ICD codes provide a standard language of disability in young children. *J Clin Epidemiol*. 59(4):365–373.

Simeonsson RJ (2000) Early childhood intervention: toward a universal manifesto. *Infants Young Child*. 12(3):4–9.

Simeonsson RJ (2009) ICF-CY: A universal tool for documentation of disability. *Journal of Policy and Practise in Intellectual Disabilities*. 6(2) 70–72.

Simonian S (2006) Screening and identification in pediatric primary care. *Behav Modif*. 30:114–131.

Singhania R, Sonksen P (2004) The Indian picture puzzle test – a developmental test designed and standardised for Indian children. *Indian J Pediatr*. 71(5): 387–396.

Song J, Zhu YM, Gu XY (1982) Restandardization of Denver Developmental Screening Test for Shanghai children. *Chin Med J (Engl)*. 95(5):375–380.

Sonnander K (2000) Early identification of children with developmental disabilities. *Acta Paediatr*. (Suppl) 89(434):17–23.

Sparrow SS, Balla DA, Cicchetti DV (1984) *Vineland Adaptive Behavior Scales*. Circle Pines, American Guidance Service.

Spiker D, Hebbeler K, Mallik S (2005) Developing and implementing early intervention programs for children with established disabilities. In: Guralnick MJ, ed. *The developmental systems approach to early intervention*. Baltimore, MD: Paul H Brookes Publishing Co: 305–351.

Spiker D et al. (1991) Design issues in a randomized clinical trial of a behavioral intervention: insights from the Infant Health and Development Program. *J Dev Behav Pediatr*. 12(6):386–393.

Srinath S et al. (2005) Epidemiological study of child & adolescent psychiatric disorders in urban and rural areas of Bangalore, India. *Indian J Med Res*. 122(1):67–79.

Sriyaporn PP, Pissasoontorn W, Sakdisawadi O (1994) Denver Developmental Screening Test survey of Bangkok children. *Asia Pac J Public Health*. 7(3):173–177.

Srsen KG, Vidmar G, Zupan A (2005) Applicability of the pediatric evaluation of disability inventory in Slovenia. *J Child Neurol*. 20(5): 411–416.

Starfield BH et al. (1976) Continuity and coordination in primary care: their achievement and utility. *Med Care*. 14(7):625–636.

Stein RE (2004) Measurement of children's health. *Ambul Pediatr*. 4 (4 Suppl):365–370.

Stein RE, Silver EJ (1999) Operationalizing a conceptually based noncategorical definition: a first look at US children with chronic conditions. *Arch Pediatr Adolesc Med*. 153(1): 68–74.

Stein Z, Belmont L, Durkin M (1987) Mild mental retardation and severe mental retardation compared: experiences in eight less developed countries. *Ups J Med Sci Suppl*. 44:89–96.

Stern D (1998) Mothers' emotional needs. *Pediatrics*. 102:1250–1252.

Stier DM et al. (1993) Are children born to young mothers at increased risk for maltreatment? *Pediatrics*. 91:642–648.

Sturmey P et al. (1992) Portage guide to early intervention: cross-cultural aspects and intra-cultural variability. *Child Care Health Dev*. 18(6): 377–394.

Sun XB et al. (2003) [Study on the disabilities in aged 0–7 years children in Shenzhen, China.] *Zhonghua Liu Xing Bing Xue Za Zhi*. 24(11):1016–1019 (in Chinese).

Super CM, Herrera MG, Mora JO (1990) Long-term effects of food supplementation and psychosocial intervention on the physical growth of Colombian infants at risk of malnutrition. *Child Dev*. 61(1):29–49.

Swailem AR et al. (1988) Perinatal mortality in a Saudi maternity hospital. *Acta Paediatr Scand*. 346 (supplement):57–69.

Swick KJ, Williams RD (2006) An analysis of Bronfenbrenner's bio ecological perspective for early childhood educators: implications for working with families experiencing stress. *Early Childhood Education Journal*. 33(5): 371–378.

Taylor HG et al. (1998) Predictors of early school age outcomes in very low birth weight children. *J Dev Behav Pediatr.* 19(4):235–243.

Teferra T (2003) Early intervention practices: Ethiopia. In: Odom SL et al. eds. *Early intervention practices around the world.* Baltimore: Paul H. Brookes: 91–111

Teutsch C (2003) Patient-doctor communication. *Med Clin North Am.* 87(5):1115–1145.

Theeranate K, Chuengchitraks S (2005) Parent's Evaluation of Developmental Status (PEDS) detects developmental problems compared to Denver II. *J Med Assoc Thai.* 88(Suppl3):S188–192.

Thomasgard M, Metz WP (2004) Promoting child social-emotional growth in primary care settings: using a developmental approach. *Clin Pediatr (Phila).* 43(2):119–127.

Thorburn M et al. (1992) Identification of childhood disability in Jamaica: the 'ten questions' screen. *Int J Rehabil Res.* 15:115–127.

Thorburn MJ (2003) Paraprofessionals in low-cost early intervention programs: Jamaica. In: Odom SL et al. eds. *Early intervention practices around the world.* Baltimore: Paul H. Brookes: 191–213.

Tirosh E, Amit Y, Harel J (1999) The psychologist's role in a child development centre. The therapist's perceptions. *Int J Rehabil Res.* 22(2):147–150.

Tombokan-Runtukahu J, Nitko AJ (1992) Translation, cultural adjustment, and validation of a measure of adaptive behavior. *Res Dev Disabil.* 13:481–501.

Trani JF (2009) Screening children for disability. *Lancet.* 374(9704):1806–1807.

Treffers P (2002) *Issues in adolescent health and development: Adolescent pregnancy.* Geneva, World Health Organization.

Trotman H, Barton M (2005) The impact of the establishment of a neonatal intensive care unit on the outcome of very low birthweight infants at the University Hospital of the West Indies. *West Indian Med J.* 54(5):297–301.

Tsai-Hsing Hsia S, McCabe H, Jen Li B (2003) Cultural issues and service provision in rural areas: People's Republic of China. In: Odom SL et al., eds. *Early intervention practices around the world.* Baltimore: Paul H. Brookes: 27–49.

Tulloch J (1999) Integrated approach to child health in developing countries. *Lancet.* 354 (Suppl 2):SII16–20.

Tunstill J et al. (2005) Sure Start local programmes: implications of case study data from the national evaluation of Sure Start. *Children and Society.* 19(2):158–171.

Turmusani M, Vreede A, Wirz SL (2002) Some ethical issues in community-based rehabilitation initiatives in developing countries. *Disabil Rehabil.* 24(10):558–564.

Udwin O, Yule W (1982) Validational data on Lowe and Costello's Symbolic Play Test. *Child Care Health Dev.* 8(6): 361–366.

Ueda R (1978) Standardization of the Denver Developmental Screening Test on Tokyo children. *Dev Med Child Neurol.* 20(5):647–656.

UNICEF (2004) Low birth weight: country, regional and global estimates., United Nations Children's Fund and World Health Organization, New York.

United Nations (2006) *United Nations Convention on the Rights of Persons with Disabilities.* New York (http://www.un.org/disabilities/default.asp?navid=12&pid=150 accessed 22.8.2009)

United Nations (1989) *United Nations Convention on the Rights of the Child.* United Nations General Assembly Document A/RES/44/25. New York (http://www.un.org/documents/ga/res/44/a44r025.htm ; accessed 10.12.2008)

United Nations (1993) *The Standard Rules on the Equalization of Opportunities for Persons with Disabilities.* Resolution 48/96 adopted by the United Nations General Assembly, 48th session, 20 December 1993. New York (http://www.un.org/esa/socdev/enable/dissre00.htm ; accessed 22.08.2009).

US Department of Health and Human Services (2002) *The impacts of Early Head Start.* A detailed guide for administration for children and families. Making a difference in the lives of infants and toddlers and their families. Washington, DC.

van Widenfelt BM et al. (2005) Translation and cross-cultural adaptation of assessment instruments used in psychological research with children and families. *Clin Child Fam Psychol Rev.* 8(2):135–147.

Vanderbilt-Adriance E, Shaw DS (2006) Neighborhood risk and the development of resilience. *Ann N Y Acad Sci.* 1094:359–362.

Vazir S, Kashinath K (1999) Influence of ICDS on psychosocial development of rural children in Southern India. *Journal of the Indian Academy of Applied Psychology.* 11–24.

Vazir S et al. (1994a) A comparison of Indian and American Scales of Child Development. *Journal of the Indian Academy of Applied Psychology.* 20: 175–181.

Vazir S et al. (1994b) Screening test battery for assessment of psychosocial development. *Indian Pediatrics.* 31: 1465–1475.

REFERENCES

Vega J et al. (1999) Chronic exposure to environmental lead in Chilean infants. II: Effects on the psychomotor development. *Rev Med Chil.* 127(1):28–37.

Venter A (1997a) Caregivers' expectations of services at Baragwanath Hospital, Soweto and their understanding of the child's disability. *Dev Med Child Neurol.*39(12):815–820.

Venter A (1997b) Developmental paediatrics – the coming of age? *S Afr Med J.* 87(12):1664–1665.

Verma IC, Prema A, Puri RK (1992) Health effects of consanguinity in Pondichery. *Indian Pediatr.* 29(6):685–692.

Volpe JJ (1997) Brain injury in the premature infant: neuropathology, clinical aspects, and pathogenesis. *Ment Retard and Dev Disabil.* 3:3–12.

Vos-Vromans DC, Ketelaar M, Gorter JW (2005) Responsiveness of evaluative measures for children with cerebral palsy: the Gross Motor Function Measure and the Pediatric Evaluation of Disability Inventory. *Disabil Rehabil.* 27(20): 1245–1252.

Wachs TD et al. (1993) Relations between nutrition and cognitive performance in Egyptian toddlers. *Intelligence.* 17(2): 151–172.

Wachs TD et al. (2005) Maternal education and intelligence predict offspring diet and nutritional status. *J Nutr.* 135:2179–2186.

Walker SP et al. (2005) Effects of early childhood psychosocial stimulation and nutritional supplementation on cognition and education in growth-stunted Jamaican children: prospective cohort study. *Lancet.* 366(9499):1804–1807.

Walker SP et al. (2006) Effects of psychosocial stimulation and dietary supplementation in early childhood on psychosocial functioning in late adolescence: follow-up of randomised controlled trial. *BMJ.* 333(7566):472.

Walker SP et al. (2007) Child development: risk factors for adverse outcomes in developing countries. *Lancet.* 369(9556):145–157.

Wasserman GA et al. (1990) Psychosocial attributes and life experiences of minority mothers: age and ethnic variations. *Child Dev.* 61: 566–580.

Wechsler D (1991) *Manual for the Wechsler Intelligence Scale for Children*, 3rd ed. San Antonio, TX: The Psychological Corporation(WISC-III).

Weitzman CC, Leventhal JM (2006) Screening for behavioral health problems in primary care. *Curr Opin Pediatr.* 18(6):641–648.

Weitzman CC et al. (2004) More evidence for reach out and read: a home-based study. *Pediatrics.* 113(5):1248–1253.

Wendland-Carro J, Piccinini CA, Millar WS (1999) The role of an early intervention on enhancing the quality of mother-infant interaction. *Child Dev.* 70(3):713–721.

Were FN, Bwibo NO (2006) Two year neurological outcomes of very low birth weight infants. *East Afr Med J.* 83(5):243–249.

Werner EE (1992) The children of Kauai: resiliency and recovery in adolescence and adulthood. *J Adolesc Health.* 13:262–268.

Whaley SE et al. (1998) Infant predictors of cognitive development in an undernourished Kenyan population. *J Dev Behav Pediatr.* 19(3):169–177.

WHO (1992) *The ICD-10 Classification of Mental and Behavioural Disorders: clinical descriptions and diagnostic guidelines.*Geneva, World Health Organization.

WHO (1998a) *Postpartum care of the mother and newborn: a practical guide.* Geneva, World Health Organization (http://www.who.int/reproductive-health/publications/msm_98_3/index.html).

WHO (1998b) *Improving mother-child interaction to promote better psychosocial development in children.* Geneva, World Health Organization (WHO/MSA/MHP/98.1)

WHO (1999) *A critical link: interventions for physical growth and psychological development. A review.* Geneva, World Health Organization (WHO/CHS/CAH/99–3).

WHO (2001a) *Integrated Management of Childhood Illness. Counsel the mother on feeding, care for development, when to return and the mother's health.* Geneva, World Health Organization.

WHO (2001b) *International Classification of Functioning, Disability and Health.* Geneva, World Health Organization.

WHO (2001c) IMCI *Care for Child Development.* Geneva, World Health Organization (http://www.who.int/child_adolescent_health/documents/imci_care_for_development/en/index.html; accessed 17 October 2008).

WHO (2003) *Shaping the future: the World Health Report 2003.* Geneva: World Health Organization.

WHO (2004a) *International Statistical Classification of Diseases and Related Health Problems*, Tenth Revision, World Health Organization. Second Edition. Geneva, World Health Organization.

WHO (2004b) Atlas: Country Resources for Neurological Disorders. Geneva, World Health Organization. Geneva,World Health Organization.

WHO (2005a) Mental Health Atlas. Geneva, World Health Organization.

WHO (2005b) WHO AIMS: Mental Health Systems in low- and middle-income countries: a WHO-AIMS cross-national analysis. Geneva, World Health Organization.

WHO (2005c) Atlas: Child and adolescent mental health resources: Global concerns, implications for the future. Geneva, World Health Organization.

WHO (2005d) Atlas: Epilepsy care in the world. Geneva, World Health Organization.

WHO (2006a) *Anti-retroviral therapy of HIV infection in infants and children in resource-limited settings: towards universal access, Recommendations for a public health approach.* Geneva, World Health Organization (http://www.who.int/hiv/pub/vct/hivstaging/en/index.html ; accessed 21 August 2008).

WHO (2006b) *Mental retardation: from knowledge to action.* New Delhi, WHO Regional Office for South-East Asia (http://www.searo.who.int/en/Section1174/Section1199/Section1567/Section1825_8090.htm accessed September 26, 2007).

WHO (2007a) *International Classification of Functioning, Disability and Health for Children and Youth* (ICF-CY). Geneva, World Health Organization.

WHO (2007b) Atlas: Global resources for persons with intellectual disabilities

WHO (2010) *Community based rehabilitation guidelines.* Geneva, World Health Organization.

Whitt JK, Casey PH (1982) The mother infant relationship and infant development: the effect of pediatric intervention. *Child Dev.* 53(4):948–956.

Wijnhoven TM et al. (2004) Assessment of gross motor development in the WHO Multicentre Growth Reference Study. *Food Nutr Bull.* 25(1Suppl):S37–45.

Williams J et al. (2004) Diagnosis and treatment of behavioral health disorders in pediatric practice. *Pediatrics.* 114:601–606.

Williams PD (1984) The Metro-Manila Developmental Screening Test: a normative study. *Nurs Res.* 33(4):208–212.

Wirz S et al. (2005) Field testing of the ACCESS materials: a portfolio of materials to assist health workers to identify children with disabilities and offer simple advice to mothers. *Int J Rehabil Res.* 28 (4):293–302.

Wolf MJ et al. (1997) Neurodevelopmental outcome in babies with a low Apgar score from Zimbabwe. *Dev Med Child Neurol.* 39(12): 821–826.

Wolf MJ et al. (1999) Neurodevelopmental outcome at 1 year in Zimbabwean neonates with extreme hyperbilirubinaemia. *Eur J Pediatr.* 158(2):111–114.

Wyman PA et al. (1999) Caregiving and developmental factors differentiating young at-risk urban children showing resilient versus stress-affected outcomes: a replication and extension. *Child Dev.* 70(3):645–659.

Yalaz K, Epir S (1983) The Denver Developmental Screening Test: normative data for Ankara children. *Turk J Pediatr.* 25(4):245–258.

Yang TF et al. (2003) Effect of botulinum toxin type A on cerebral palsy with upper limb spasticity. *Am J Phys Med Rehabil.* 82(4):284–289.

Yaqoob M et al. (2004) Mild intellectual disability in children in Lahore, Pakistan: aetiology and risk factors. *J Intellect Disabil Res.* 48(7):663–671.

Yaqoob M et al. (1993) Early child health in Lahore, Pakistan: II. Inbreeding. *Acta Paediatr.* 390 (suppl.):17–26.

Young A et al. (2008) Disabled children (0–3 years) and integrated services – the impact of Early Support. *Health Soc Care Community.* 16(3):222–233.

Young HB et al. (1982) Milk and lactation: some social and developmental correlates among 1,000 infants. *Pediatrics.* 69(2): 169–175.

Youssef RM et al. (2002) Correlates of unintended pregnancy in Beheira governorate, Egypt. *East Mediterr Health J.* 8(4–5):521–536.

Yunis K et al. (2003) Low socioeconomic status and neonatal outcomes in an urban population in a developing country. *J Matern Fetal Neonatal Med.* 14(5):338.

Zeanah CH, ed. (2000) *Handbook of infant mental health*, 2nd ed. New York: Guilford Press.

Zero to Three (2005) *Diagnostic classification of mental health and developmental disorders of infancy and early childhood: revised edition (DC: 0–3R).* Washington, DC.

Zigler E, Styfco SJ (2004) *Head Start debates.* Baltimore: Brookes Pub Co.

Zinkin P, McConachie H, eds (1995). *Disabled children and developing countries*, London: MacKeith Press (Clinics in Developmental Medicine No. 136).

Zuckerman B, Augustyn M, Parker S (2001) Child development in pediatrics: beyond rhetoric. *Arch Pediatr Adolesc Med.* 155(12):1294–1295.

Zuckerman B et al. (1997) The Healthy Steps for young children program. *Zero to Three.* 17(6):20–25.

Zuckerman B et al. (2004a) Healthy Steps: a case study of innovation in pediatric practice. *Pediatrics.* 114(3):820–826.

Zuckerman B et al. (2004b) Prevalence and correlates of high-quality basic pediatric preventive care. *Pediatrics.* 114:1522–1529.

Annex 1

World Health Organization Survey
Care for young children with developmental difficulties

Dear ……………………………………,

We have identified you as a key expert on children with developmental difficulties in your country. We request your participation in this survey, which is part of a comprehensive review commissioned by the World Health Organization to help countries and international organizations to prevent and manage developmental risks and difficulties in children from birth to 3 years of age. Our goal is to identify the global need of systems and services for young children at risk for or with developmental difficulties. This survey is being sent to ONE expert from each country.

The survey consists of 30 questions and will take approximately 1 hour of your time. We understand there may be difficulties in providing answers to specific questions in situations where there is no official information available and/or there may be marked variability in resources available in various parts of the same country. We would appreciate it if you consult references or informants when possible but when this is not possible we would be grateful if you could provide your *best estimate* for the questions. Data will be compiled and reported as a whole and your name will be kept confidential. We will acknowledge your contribution in the final review if you indicate this at the end of this survey. Please indicate on the survey your preferred long term contact information. As a gift, we would like to send you a package of documents related to the field and would also like to keep in touch with you in other international initiatives related to child development.

We would like to encourage you to complete the survey by clicking on the web link below:

https://fs10.formsite.com/ertemilgi/form502944769/form_login.html

This site is user friendly and enables you to create your own account and password so that you can save and return to your results at any time. Alternatively, you may contact Dr. Ilgi Ertem to receive an attachment of the survey. Please complete and return survey before March 15th, 2007. Please contact Dr. Ilgi Ertem by e-mail if you have questions.

We thank you in advance for your time and all your efforts, and hope that the results of this survey and the final report will help ensure a better future for children and their families.

World Health Organization
Department of Child and Adolescent Health and Development

Meena Cabral de Mello
Senior Scientist Department of Child and
 Adolescent Health and Development Family
 and Community Health Cluster World
 Health Organization
Avenue Appia 20 CH-1211 Geneva 27
Tel: (41 22) 791 3616 (41 22) 791 4239
Fax: (41 22) 791 4853
E-mail: cabraldemellom@who.int

Ilgi Ertem M.D.
Associate Professor of Pediatrics
Developmental-Behavioral Pediatrics Unit
Ankara University School of Medicine
Cebeci, Ankara, 06100 Turkey
Visiting Professor at Yale University Department
 of Pediatrics
New Haven, CT, USA
Tel: 203-688-2468 (work)
Fax: 203-785-3932
E-mail: ertemilgi@yahoo.com

Definitions of terms used throughout survey

Please review the definitions below of terms used throughout the survey before you complete the survey. The following terms, listed in alphabetical order below, are written in italics throughout the survey.

Caregiver: An adult (parent, family member or other) who parents, takes care of child.

Child development: All areas of development including cognitive, language, emotional, behavioral, social, fine and gross motor development.

Developmental difficulty: Signs and symptoms of arrest, alteration, delay, disability in any developmental area including cognitive, language, emotional, behavioral, social, fine and gross motor difficulties.

Developmental risk: Biological and psychosocial conditions that pose risks to optimal development. Biological risks include conditions such as premature birth, low birth weight, malnutrition, infectious diseases, and genetic disorders. Psychosocial risks include conditions such as poverty, maternal depression, child-caregiver interaction problems, caregiver illness and/or stress, human discrimination, violence, war, natural disaster. Developmental risks may be multiple and combined. A child with a risk may not yet demonstrate difficulty or delay.

Early intervention (EI) services: Any continuous service provided by specifically trained people aimed at helping the child's cognitive (intellectual), social or emotional development.

Physical rehabilitation therapy (PT): Any intervention aiming to remedy disabilities affecting a child's difficulties in motor development.

Provider: Trained person providing health, educational or other services for child and/or caregivers to address developmental difficulties.

Young child: Child aged 0–36 months.

ANNEX 1

WHO SURVEY
Care for young children with developmental difficulties

Section 1.
Information about respondent

Country surveyed:
....
Name of respondent:
....
Title and current position:
....
Address of the institution in which you work:
....

....

....
E-mail:
....
Telephone: Fax:
....

Is this your country of origin?
a) Yes
b) If no, then how many years have you lived in this country? .... years.

Please indicate your primary discipline (*check one only*):
☐ a) General pediatrician
☐ b) Pediatric neurologist
☐ c) Developmental or developmental-behavioral pediatrician
☐ d) Other medical/doctor (indicate field if other than general practitioner):
     ....
☐ e) Psychiatrist
☐ f) Psychologist
☐ g) Educator/teacher
☐ h) Social worker
☐ i) Nurse
☐ j) Other (*please describe*): ....

How many years of experience do you have in working with young children with *developmental risks*, delays, disabilities or *difficulties*? (*check one only*):
☐ a) Less than 1 year
☐ b) 1–5 years
☐ c) 6–10 years
☐ d) 11–15 years
☐ e) Greater than 15 years

In what ways have you been involved with children with *developmental difficulties* (*check all that apply*):
- ☐ a) Academic (teaching in schools/universities)
- ☐ b) Clinical service
- ☐ c) Research
- ☐ d) Administrative
- ☐ e) Advocacy
- ☐ f) Policy maker within government
- ☐ g) Non-profit organization
- ☐ h) Other (please describe): ....

Section 2.
Role of health care *providers* in the prevention of *developmental difficulties*.

1. In your country how far are most villages/towns/communities from trained health care *providers*? (*check one only*):
   - ☐ a) Within walking distance
   - ☐ b) Accessible by transportation that is affordable to most of the population
   - ☐ c) Not accessible by transportation that is affordable to most of the population
   - ☐ d) Other (please describe): ....

2. Who do most young children see for their healthcare? *Please check X in one box (a–e) for each question (2.1–2.3). Healthcare provider in this question indicates anyone other than a medical doctor, such as a nurse, midwife or other trained healthcare provider.*

	a) Mostly same medical doctor	b) Mostly different medical doctors	c) Mostly same healthcare provider	d) Mostly different healthcare provider	e) Other (please explain)
2.1 Primary-preventive healthcare (immunizations, growth monitoring, nutritional counseling)					
2.2 Acute healthcare (healthcare when children have an acute illness such as diarrhea, respiratory tract infection)					
2.3 Chronic illness (malnutrition, asthma, HIV-AIDS, developmental difficulty)					

3. Please indicate if the following trained *providers* exist? If they exist, are there a sufficient number of them to serve **more than 50% of all *young children* in need of their services**. *Check X in one box for each provider.*

Trained providers	Don't exist	Exist Sufficient	Exist Insufficient
3.1 Primary healthcare doctors, general practitioners			
3.2 Primary healthcare nurses			
3.3 Home visitors with background in healthcare			
3.4 Home visitors with background in discipline other than healthcare			
3.5 Home visiting volunteers			
3.6 Pediatricians			
3.7 Pediatric neurologists			
3.8 Developmental-behavioral pediatricians			

ANNEX 1

Trained providers	Don't exist	Exist Sufficient	Exist Insufficient
3.9 Child psychiatrists			
3.10 Professionals trained specifically in infant mental health			
3.11 Child psychologists			
3.12 Early intervention/early childhood development specialists			
3.13 Special education teachers			
3.14 Pediatric physiotherapists			
3.15 Pediatric occupational therapists			
3.16 Child speech and language therapists			
3.17 Social workers trained to work with children and families			
3.18 Child care (day care, nursery school) teachers			

4. What proportion of **all primary healthcare *providers*** (doctors and other healthcare *providers*) **have the expertise and training to provide** the services listed? *Check X in one box for each question.*

What proportion of primary healthcare providers in your country know how to:	Most (100–75%)	Many (74–50%)	Some (49–25%)	Few (24–5%)	Very few–none (4–0%)
4.1 Use interview and observational skills to identify *biologic developmental risk* factors (such as low birth weight) in *young children*					
4.2 Use interview and observational skills to assess *social-emotional developmental risk* factors (such as maternal depression) in *young children*					
4.3 Use interview and observational skills to assess the all aspects of a *young child's development*					
4.4 Use standardized validated instruments to assess the *development* of *young children*					
4.5 Use standardized methods to assess malnutrition in *young children*					
4.6 Use interview and observation skills to assess if a child has cerebral palsy in the first year of life					
4.7 Use interview and observation skills to assess if a child has autism in the first three years of life					
4.8 Assess hearing loss in the first 6 months of life					
4.9 Use interview and observational skills to assess language difficulties (apart from hearing loss) in the first 2 years of life					
4.10 Use interview and observational skills to identify difficulties in caregiver-child relationship					
4.11 Use interview and observational skills to identify child neglect and abuse					
4.12 Counsel caregivers about how to enhance the child's development (e.g., learning, communication, mental health)					
4.13 Counsel caregivers of young children with developmental risks and difficulties about how to access early intervention and rehabilitation resources					
4.14 Manage the special healthcare needs of children with developmental difficulties					

5. Are there programs that train **at least 50% of all primary healthcare providers serving children** about the types of **services listed in question 4** that help prevent and manage developmental difficulties in young children? (*Please check one only*)
   - ☐ a) Training programs do not exist
   - ☐ b) Pre-service (in schools/before graduation/starting work) training programs exists
   - ☐ c) In-service (during work) training programs exist
   - ☐ d) Both pre-service and in-service training programs exist
   - ☐ e) Other (*please describe*): ....

6. Please indicate what proportion of **all young children** in the country receive the services listed. *Please also indicate whether these services are free of charge (paid by government or other insurance and free/or minimal cost to families). A service may be received by few children but may be a free-of-charge service.*

Services	What proportion of ALL *young children* receives service?					Free of charge?	
	Most (100–75%)	Many (74–50%)	Some (49–25%)	Few (24–5%)	Very few–none (4–0%)	Yes	No
6.1 Prenatal and antenatal primary health care for mothers							
6.2 Delivery by trained birth attendants							
6.3 Primary healthcare in the first three years of life							
6.4 Continuous healthcare by the same health care provider in the first three years of life							
6.5 Prenatal screening for Down syndrome							
6.6 Neonatal screening for phenylketonuria							
6.7 Neonatal screening for hypothyroidism							
6.8 Neonatal screening for hearing loss							
6.9 Growth monitoring							
6.10 Nutritional counseling							
6.11 Iron supplementation to prevent anemia							
6.12 Iodized salt							
6.13 Basic immunizations							
6.14 Developmental surveillance (child development is followed during routine healthcare by trained providers)							
6.15 Developmental screening (standardized instruments or tests are used to detect developmental delay)							
6.16 Counseling to the caregivers during health care visits on how to enhance their child's development							
6.17 Home visiting by healthcare providers							

7. Which systems in your country are responsible for **routine home visiting**? *Check systems only if they aim to reach all **young children** in the country.*
   - ☐ a) Routine home visiting is not a part of any system
   - ☐ b) Health care system
   - ☐ c) Education system
   - ☐ d) Social services system
   - ☐ e) Other (please explain): ....

8. Who does routine home visits for **most** *young children*? *(Please check one)*
   - ☐ a) Home visiting is not a routine part of any system
   - ☐ b) Healthcare *providers*
   - ☐ c) Paid people other than healthcare providers
   - ☐ d) Non-paid volunteers
   - ☐ e) Other (please describe): ....

9. What is generally provided during home visits? *(Check all that apply)*
   - ☐ a) Immunizations
   - ☐ b) Assessment of child's growth
   - ☐ c) Assessment of all areas of *child development*
   - ☐ d) Assessment of selected areas of child development, please indicate which area:
     ....
   - ☐ e) Assessment of caregiver/family stressors and needs
   - ☐ f) Counseling caregivers about child's physical health
   - ☐ g) Counseling caregivers about how to enhance their child's development
   - ☐ h) Other (please describe): ....

Section 3.
Services for children with developmental risk and difficulties

10. In your country is there a law that mandates that young children with developmental difficulties should have access to early intervention services?
    - ☐ a) No
    - ☐ b) Yes and the law was first established in the year ....

11. Please name instruments for *developmental screening* or assessment that are used routinely in your country **by many (at least 50%) of health care *providers*** that work with children to determine the presence of *developmental difficulties in young children*.
    - ☐ a) Instruments are not used routinely
    - ☐ b) Instruments used routinely are:
      - i.   ....
      - ii. ....
      - iii. ....

12. Please name classification systems (eg: International Classification of Functioning, Diagnostic Classification 0-3) that are used in your country **by many (at least 50%) of health care *providers*** that work with children to diagnose or determine the presence of *developmental difficulties* in *young children*.
    - ☐ a) Classification systems are not routinely used
    - ☐ b) Classification systems routinely used are:
      - i.   ....
      - ii. ....
      - iii. ....

13. In the past ten years in your country have there been any population surveys that provide **specific information on the number of children aged 0–36 months** with *developmental difficulties*?
    - ☐ a) Surveys don't exist or existing surveys do not provide this specific information
    - ☐ b) Surveys provide information and the proportion of children aged 0–36 months with developmental difficulties is .... %.

14. Who is **most likely to first recognize** that a young child has developmental difficulties? (*Check one only*)
    - ☐ a) Caregivers (parents and relatives)
    - ☐ b) Pediatrician
    - ☐ c) Community medical doctor
    - ☐ d) Community healthcare provider other than medical doctor
    - ☐ e) Daycare teacher
    - ☐ f) Other (*please explain*): ....

15. Who **most often conducts** an evaluation and diagnose the child to have a developmental difficulty? (*Check one only*)
    - ☐ a) Pediatrician
    - ☐ b) Community medical doctor
    - ☐ c) Community healthcare provider other than medical doctor
    - ☐ d) Early intervention specialist
    - ☐ e) Daycare teacher
    - ☐ f) Other (*please explain*): ....

16. Who **most often decides** which kind of early intervention (EI) and/or rehabilitation services the child should receive? (*Check one only*)
    - ☐ a) Services don't exist
    - ☐ b) Pediatrician
    - ☐ c) Community medical doctor
    - ☐ d) Community healthcare provider other than medical doctor
    - ☐ e) Early intervention specialist
    - ☐ f) Daycare teacher
    - ☐ g) Other (*please explain*): ....

17. Does the child need criteria, disability score, ratio or classification to be eligible for EI and/or rehabilitation services?
    - ☐ a) Services don't exist
    - ☐ b) No
    - ☐ c) Yes, please describe what criteria make a child eligible for services:
      ....

18. What is the background training of people that provide EI in your country? (*Check one only*)
    - ☐ a) University or college level in early intervention or related discipline
    - ☐ b) High school level with focus on early intervention or related discipline
    - ☐ c) One-two years of specific training in EI or related discipline
    - ☐ d) Less than 1 year but more than 1 month of specific training in EI or related discipline
    - ☐ e) One month or less of specific training
    - ☐ f) Other ....

19. In your country how are EI services most commonly provided? (*Check one only*)
    - ☐ a) Home based services to individual child
    - ☐ b) Center based services to individual child
    - ☐ c) Center based services to groups of children
    - ☐ d) Other (*please describe*): ....

20. In your country, are caregivers/families generally present during EI hours? (*Check one only*)
    - ☐ a) Caregivers are present during most EI hours
    - ☐ b) Caregivers are not present during most EI hours
    - ☐ c) Other (*please describe*): ....

21. In your country, how are EI services usually provided?
    - ☐ a) EI is mostly family centered (caregivers are viewed as an active partner and have equal input as professionals)
    - ☐ b) EIS are mostly child centered (caregivers are informed but professionals mainly focus on improving skills of child)
    - ☐ c) Other: ....

22. Are young children with developmental difficulties placed in residential centers (centers where children live for long periods without family) in your country?
    - ☐ a) Residential centers for young children do not exist
    - ☐ b) Residential centers exist and approximately .... % of young children with developmental difficulties live in residential centers

23. Please indicate what proportion of **all young children** with *developmental difficulties* or their **families** receive the services listed in your country. Please also indicate whether these services are free of charge (government subsidized or otherwise insured) and at minimal cost to families for **all young children** who are in need of these services.

Services	What proportion of all *young children* with developmental difficulties or their families receive services?					Free of charge?	
	Most (100–75%)	Many (74–50%)	Some (49–25%)	Few (24–5%)	Very few–none (4–0%)	Yes	No
23.1 EI if the young child has developmental delay							
23.2 EI if the young child is not delayed but is at risk of developmental delay due to biological causes such as premature birth or malnutrition							
23.3 EI if the young child is **not yet delayed but is at risk of developmental delay** due to psychosocial causes such as poverty or maternal depression							
23.4 Psychological counseling							
23.5 Information to caregivers on how to help the child develop							
23.6 *Physical rehabilitation* for motor development							
23.7 Orthopedic treatments							
23.8 EI for cognitive difficulties							
23.9 EI for social and or emotional difficulties							
23.10 EI for difficulties in caregiver-child relationship							

Services	What proportion of all *young children* with developmental difficulties or their families receive services?					Free of charge?	
	Most (100–75%)	Many (74–50%)	Some (49–25%)	Few (24–5%)	Very few– none (4–0%)	Yes	No
23.11 Occupational therapy for fine motor difficulties							
23.12 Hearing aids							
23.13 Speech and language therapy							
23.14 Day care (child care)							
23.15 Special transportation services to reach EI							
23.16 Financial aid to caregivers for having a child with difficulties							

23.17 Please list any additional services (apart from those listed in question 23.1–23.16) that young children and their families may be likely to receive in your country:

....
....
....
....
....

24. In your country what is the major source of funding for services listed in questions 23.1–23.17?
   - ☐ a) Government
   - ☐ b) Non-profit organizations (NGOs)
   - ☐ c) For profit organizations
   - ☐ d) Caregiver's funds
   - ☐ e) Other (*please describe*): ....

25. What kind of impact do the following circumstances have in obstructing or facilitating the access of children who need the services you have listed in question 23. *Please check X in one box for each question 24.1–24.10.*

	No impact	Some impact	Great impact
25.1 Maternal education			
25.2 Paternal education			
25.3 Caregivers income			
25.4 Geographical location in country			
25.5 Urban (city) or rural (countryside, village) location			
25.6 Ethnicity			
25.7 Religion			
25.8 Stigmatization (e.g.: child may not be allowed to enter nursery schools)			